THE NO NEED TO DIET BOOK

Plantbased Pixie is a nutritionist (MSc) (AfN), award-winning food blogger, writer and speaker. She has also been featured at many events, in various publications and on BBC World News and Channel 5 as a nutritional expert.

www.plantbased-pixie.com
www.pixieturnernutrition.com

ALSO BY PIXIE TURNER

The Wellness Rebel

THE No Need to DIET BOOK

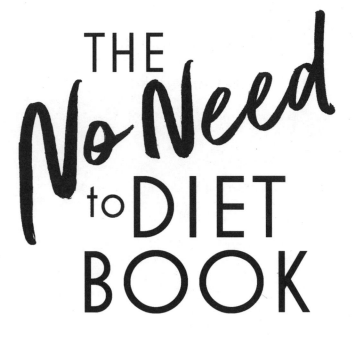

PIXIE TURNER

HEAD
of ZEUS

An Anima Book

This is an Anima book, first published in the UK in 2019 by
Head of Zeus Ltd

9 7 5 3 1 2 4 6 8

A catalogue record for this book is available from
the British Library.

ISBN (HB): 9781788547154
ISBN (E): 9781788547178

Printed and bound in Great Britain by
CPI Group (UK) Ltd, Croydon CRO 4YY

Head of Zeus Ltd
5–8 Hardwick Street
London EC1R 4RG
WWW.HEADOFZEUS.COM

CONTENTS

To all the researchers, activists, and healthcare professionals
who came before me and made this possible

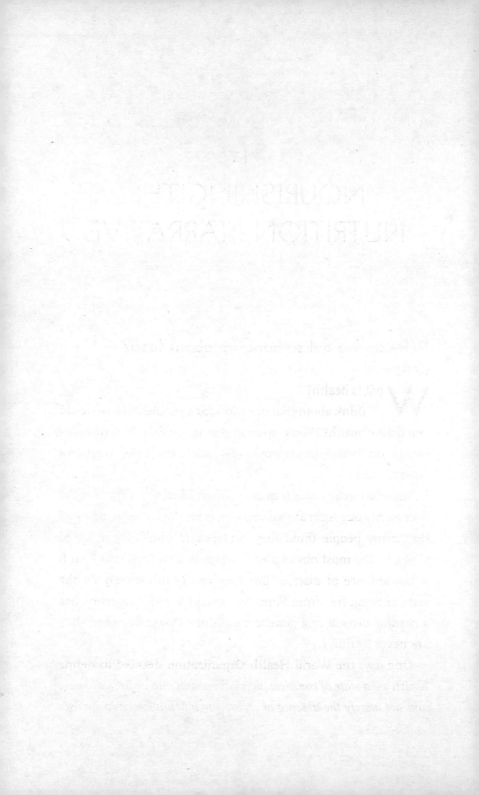

1
NOURISHING THE NUTRITION NARRATIVE

Why do we get so hung up about food?

What is health?

Think about that question for a moment. How would you define health? Would you say you are healthy? How important is your health? What would you sacrifice in order to achieve good health?

These are really tough questions, and I don't think there is necessarily one right answer. Health is an elusive term, and one that many people think they understand until they're asked about it. The most obvious and common answer is that health is the absence of disease. But how can health merely be the state of being free from illness or injury? What if someone has a chronic disease or a genetic condition? Does that mean they are never healthy?

One day, the World Health Organization decided to define health as '*a state of complete physical, mental and social well-being and not merely the absence of disease or infirmity*', a step further than the 'health = no disease' idea. But this has been subject to a great deal of criticism, particularly due to the rise of chronic disease. To be in a 'complete' state of health is nigh on impossible for most people most of the time, and so this goal is quite unrealistic. Also, the WHO definition of health was set in the 1940s, which is quite some time ago, and hasn't been updated since, even though the health landscape has shifted dramatically. Whereas we used to be mostly affected by communicable diseases, like polio or smallpox, now we are faced with chronic conditions that affect people for many years of their life.

Is poor health something that always needs to be fixed? Some would argue that we have a moral responsibility to be healthy, but again, what if that's not possible? If you look anywhere in the media or to public-health initiatives, you'll see messages about how we're going through a chronic health crisis. But of course, we have an answer to pretty much all these chronic diseases: whether it's heart disease or diabetes, the answer is simple – we have too many fat people! Put them all on diets and everything will be fine!

A brief history of diets

Can you remember a time in your life without diets? Without either seeing ads about diets, hearing about diets, or being on a diet? Most of us struggle to imagine it.

I've never been on a traditional diet. Never done Weight Watchers or Slimming World or anything like that. But I have done juicing, 'clean eating', paleo, veganism, vegetarianism and even a brief attempt at raw veganism.

There are now endless diets to choose from, all with different rules and different methods. They're nothing new: diets have been around for ages, recycled over and over again into something that sounds new and exciting.

The British poet Lord Byron popularised the first 'fad diet' in the 1800s. His diet involved drinking three tablespoons of vinegar in a glass of water before a meal to aid weight loss (something that wellness took up again recently, and celebrity physician Dr Oz). The first low-carb diet book came out in the 1860s and was extremely popular. At the end of the 19th century, Horace Fletcher, an American entrepreneur, gained the nickname the 'Great Masticator', as his diet revolved around – you guessed it – chewing. You could eat as much as you liked, but each mouthful of food had to be chewed at least 100 times, by which point it would be liquid. In the 1920s, the 'flappers' became popular and so did the fashion for thin, boyish figures for women. This brought along with it the cigarette diet, diet pills, chewing gum, laxatives and contraptions that made outlandish fat-reducing claims. The idea of counting the number of calories in food only took off after American nutrutionist Dr Lulu Hunt Peters published, in 1918, *Diet & Health: With Key to the Calories*, which encouraged looking at food as calories instead, and so started the trend of eating only a certain number of calories a day. It sold millions of copies throughout the 1920s, becoming the first diet bestseller. Suddenly calories became a big deal.

Then came the Grapefruit or Hollywood diet, tapeworms (seriously?!), the popular Hay diet, Weight Watchers, and the ever-famous Cabbage Soup diet, followed by Atkins and the low-carb revolution that spanned all the way from the 1960s to the early 2000s. Meal-replacement shakes started catching on in the 1970s, which certainly paved the way for the juice and smoothie trend. Now we have weight-loss groups, veganism, low-carb, low-fat, fruitarians, carnivores, juice cleanses, intermittent fasting, detoxes – the works.

For a long period of history, food was scarce and so having more than you needed was a sign of wealth and power. But now there is so much food to go around and the power dynamic has shifted. An abundance of food is no longer desirable, so instead we prize having willpower to refuse this abundance. Thinness became power, and diets the way we sought to get there.

But diets go back far beyond the last 200 years. Humans have always been a bit weird when it comes to food. Once we reached the point where we were no longer warding off starvation, we sought additional meaning from food and eating. All of a sudden, we became more aware of the direct connection between eating and death: for us to eat and survive, something must die, whether it's plant, animal, or both. By surviving we must kill, and that feels uncomfortable. So we created rituals around death, stories about the afterlife, and we created food traditions that allow us to focus on food as celebration and enjoyment instead of death. This has the added bonus of allowing us to believe we are above other creatures; that we are not just animals – we've transcended that.

Overwhelmed by choice, by the threat of mortality that lurks behind any wrong choice, we crave rules from outside ourselves that will keep us safe. People willingly and happily hand over their freedom in exchange for the rules and restrictions that a diet offers, all for the promise of a relief from having to make choices. If you are free to choose, you risk taking full responsibility for your choices, and you can be blamed for anything that happens to you: weight gain, illness, ageing, even death. When we die, we want people to think 'But they did everything right', not 'Well, they had it coming'.

But of course, in reality, it doesn't work like this. If a diet fails, we still blame ourselves, because the diet can't be wrong if so many others have succeeded in it: we must not have done it right. And so we continue.

As Michelle Allison, Canadian registered dietitian, so beautifully put it: 'This is why arguments about diet get so vicious, so quickly. You are not merely disputing facts, you are pitting your wild gamble to avoid death against someone else's.' Diets are as personal as identity, and as powerful as religion.

Food is identity is religion

When we think of the word 'cult', we usually associate it with something religious, like Scientology. But more recently the term has been used to describe groups who share a collective viewpoint, and who define themselves by that viewpoint. In that sense, the word 'cult' describes diets perfectly. We so often define ourselves by the food we eat: we say, 'I *am* vegan', not 'I *eat* vegan'. The food we eat becomes an inherent part of our identity, which in some ways makes total sense, as the food we eat is digested and used to make up our muscles, our bones, our skin – every cell in our body. In that sense, you could argue that we really are what we eat.

Participation in a cult provides a sense of belonging: people become part of something bigger and more meaningful than themselves. It allows us to identify ourselves in relation to the whole population, identifying our similarities and differences and creating a notion of us vs them. Raw foodists, for example, eat in a way that very sharply differentiates them from the masses, but also provides a group of like-minded individuals. Food is also used to emphasise racial divides. Many ethnic slurs are based on dietary habits: Krauts for Germans; Rice Eater or Dog Eater for various Asian groups; Frogs for the French; and Limey for Brits (which originated from British sailors eating limes to ward off scurvy). Dietary beliefs unify the in-group and distinguish its members from the out-group.

More recently, 'soy boy' is now being used as a derogatory term for males who are seen as being less masculine. The idea is that if you eat soy products you are obviously weak and feminine, based on the (debunked) notion that soy products increase men's oestrogen levels. Soy is commonly eaten by vegetarians and vegans, and, of course, real men eat meat. So if you don't eat meat, you're not a real man.

Anyway, I digress; back to religion. Religions have gradually become less popular over time, while food cults and diets have become more ubiquitous. This is no coincidence. Dietary cults now replace what religion once offered by prescribing food rules and rituals. Every religion has food-related rituals, especially around fasting. Muslims fast for Ramadan, Christians give up certain foods for Lent, and the Jewish have Yom Kippur. Fasting is supposed to bring someone closer to God and reaffirm their spiritual practices. The foods someone avoids can also be a public affirmation of their religion, whether it's avoiding beef in Hinduism, pork in Islam, all meat for Seventh-Day Adventists, or alcohol in Mormonism. In addition, food is often central in religious texts: just look at the apple at the heart of the Adam and Eve story for one example. Food and appetite in religion is often linked to sins associated with lust and/or the 'pleasures of the flesh' – hence the fasting.

Food cults are arguably more appealing than ever, both because they function as a proxy for religion and because of the unprecedented cultural premium placed on health, longevity and the body. Some examples of food cults might include juicing, paleo lifestyles, superfoods, fruitarianism and wellness.

Wellness is absolutely a cult. I say that with the absolute conviction of someone who was sucked in by wellness and spat back out again. Wellness is an all-consuming identity that forces you to operate in a state of constant anxiety about whether you are 'good enough', 'healthy enough', or warding off death well enough. Have you taken your superfoods today? Did you avoid soy? Have you done your meditation? Aren't you supposed to be juicing today? Being in the wellness cult means finding other people who are also doing wellness and hanging out with them in favour of your other friends. It means buying the latest wellness book, which says the exact same thing as the one before but with a different white, thin, attractive woman on the cover smiling into her bowl of greens in a way that says, 'Yes, I know I'm amazing, wouldn't you love to be me?'

The wellness industry itself is a vast hydra-headed beast – a huge web of companies and individuals making money from all those millions of us in search of better health. And it makes a hell of a lot of money – the global industry is now believed to be worth over $3 trillion. Wellness has been boosted by the growth of social media, with devotees spreading the word via hashtags, Facebook pages and Instagram posts. The leaders of the wellness cult share their meals, their selfies and their inspirational quotes on these platforms. 'Follow us!' they say. 'We will lead you along the righteous path.' This path promises a lot, but also requires a huge level of commitment. You will be thin, you will glow, you will be clean and good, both inside and out. You must meditate and do yoga, so you can achieve calmness and enlightenment. You'll be energised, rejuvenated, pure, ward off disease, age well, and be oh so happy! You could even cure cancer, according to some wellness bloggers, such as Australians Jess Ainscough and Belle Gibson, as long as you eat 'clean' and remember to detox. So they say and so they deceive, and sometimes at great cost. In 2015, Jess Ainscough died from her cancer, and Belle Gibson not only didn't cure her cancer but never had cancer in the first place.

The power of pseudoscience

Why do people buy into dietary cults and pseudoscience? The answer to that is incredibly complicated, and will be covered in much of this book, but it's immediately clear that humans have some sort of predisposition towards cults and communities in general. Arguably, religion allowed humans to form large groups that worked together effectively with a common interest, in ways that would have been impossible otherwise. If you want to bring people together, you need a common goal and a common enemy.

Diets employ this perfectly. Dieting theology centres itself around a central object: thinness. Being thin is the goal, it is everything virtuous and good, while being fat is evil, bad and morally wrong. Diets construct a system of belief around thinness as a form of salvation. They also establish guidance on how to pursue the ultimate goal of thinness, through teachings such as eating 'good' foods and banishing 'bad' foods and doing regular exercise. Dieting has its own practices and rituals, whether that is calorie counting, macro counting, juicing, taking superfoods, tracking calories burned, or weighing yourself daily. Diet books are the religious texts that share the wisdoms of the leaders. In this way, dieting exhibits a collection of characteristics – a system of beliefs, myths, emotions, practices, rituals, rules, images, texts and symbols – that qualify as a religion.

Wellness isn't exempt from this. Wellness may use the words 'healthy' and 'unhealthy' in place of 'thin' and 'fat', but to all intents and purposes they are perceived as one and the same. 'Clean eating' is just a diet with even more moralistic language. Health is thinness. Disease is fatness. Food is 'clean' and good or 'dirty' and bad. You only have to look at the leaders of the wellness movement to confirm this: they are all thin.

Diets redefine the way dieters eat. Dieting theology assigns a moral value to food and eating that pits the 'good' foods against the 'bad' ones, whatever those might be. In veganism it pits plants against animal foods; in low-carb dogma it pits greens and meat against bread and sugar. This moralisation of food leads to cycles of guilt, echoing the guilt in religious frameworks and the need to atone for your sins.

There are several tactics employed by the leaders of food cults or dietary movements. The first of these is reciprocity – think karma, an eye for an eye, and IOUs. It makes people compelled to return the favour, as they have been granted pieces of dietary wisdom, and in return they pledge to follow the rules given. This is especially powerful when it's used by leaders of diet move-ments who are charismatic and empathetic. The leaders claim to be authorities through expertise and/or personal experiences. They claim to have been exactly where you are now – usually fat and unhealthy – and offer a solution for these problems and the pain they cause you. Just like religious leaders, many dietary leaders assert their credibility and attract a follow-ing by describing their own conversion experience from fat to thin.

Once their authority has been established, these diet leaders then ask you, the dieters, for testimonials, spreading the word of the gospel by sharing your success in achieving thinness. These success stories tend to follow the same pattern: confession followed by conversion, where they adopt the new diet, then transformation from fat to thin. The fat person is always the 'before', never the 'after'. All the while, they're expressing the values of restraint and self-discipline. Many dieters discuss their new-found perspective on life after losing weight, as if their life has been magically transformed into something wonderful and worthwhile. Or if it's wellness, then they'll also focus on how amazingly healthy they feel. Maybe their skin has improved, they're no longer bloated, or they have more energy. The concept is still the same, and although wellness claims that weight isn't the focus, weight loss is always in the testimonials. Notice how dieters and wellness followers almost never keep their eating a secret? You have to announce to the world that you are paleo, write 'vegan' in your Twitter bio, and share your food on Instagram with #cleaneating. It's that old and tired joke: How do you know if someone's a vegan? Don't worry, they'll tell you.

Dieters with transformed thin bodies embody the faith and share it with others, whereas a fat body is depicted as one that is ignorant of the gospel of weight loss, and so is considered worth less. This attitude allows people to shun fatness as being sinful and shameful, and therefore validates their own bodies in the process. Fatness is treated as a moral failure within a religion devoted to thinness.

Interestingly, within the religion of diet, it seems the more sacrifices someone makes, the more strongly they will be committed to that diet. People have a deep-rooted desire to remain consistent in their attitudes and beliefs, as this is seen as strong and stable, and avoids the negative emotions that accompany doing something that doesn't align with their beliefs. Because of this, diet cults require gestures of commitment, which tend to include banning certain foods, purchasing special food items and requesting special menus or menu items when dining out. The more sacrifices required, the bigger the commitment, and the harder it is to get away. But whether it's going to a weight-loss group in person, joining a Facebook group or following people on Instagram, being part of a group helps validate beliefs and behaviour through the power of seeing others do the same. There is then an added social pressure to go along with the group and conform to avoid being shut out and ostracised. Humans feel a powerful need to belong. And so, being ostracised can have serious and devastating effects, leading to feelings of anger and sadness: consequently, dieters often feel worse after leaving (at first), which just reaffirms the strength of the claims made by food cults.

Because of this, asking someone to turn their back on a particular way of eating, or even asking them to question their food choices, is almost like asking them to change religions. It's met with anger, denial, defensiveness and outrage. People can feel like you've insulted them if you cast doubt on their dietary choices or question the effectiveness of their diet.

Diets are arguably the new religion. But then along came wellness and said, 'Hold my beer (sorry, kombucha)!', then took it to a whole other level by putting a huge price tag on health. Behind the glowing covers of clean eating and wellness books, there is a harsh form of economic exclusion that says that someone who can't afford wheatgrass or spirulina can never be truly 'well'. But wellness, whether it wants to or not, still operates under the religion of diet culture. And diet culture affects us all. I think it's fair to say that all of us use the language of religion when talking about diets and food, or have done at some point in life. We use phrases like 'I'm converted', 'It's changed my life', 'I've been good', 'A little taste of heaven'... Even diet books have a tendency to use the word 'bible' in the title. 'Temptation', 'sinful' (come on, Slimming World uses 'syns' to categorise foods, for God's sake), 'guilty' – all these words have religious connotations. We even have 'Halo Top' low-calorie ice cream, 'conscious chocolate' and 'SoulCycle' fitness classes. Moralising and theologising food and health is now the norm.

It's also important to consider the social and cognitive motivations for believing pseudoscientific claims behind many food cults. Participating in a diet or food cult does have its benefits. For one, a fat person actively pursuing the goal of thinness is socially encouraged. Being part of such a group brings with it a feeling of acceptance and belonging. Nutritional pseudoscience and diets offer clear-cut, definitive answers about what to eat and what not to eat, whereas nutrition guidelines are complicated, nuanced, and change in the face of new evidence. Motivation for definitive answers, coupled with the social pressures of wanting to belong, are powerful tools for influencing behaviour.

The moralisation of good and bad foods – foods you can and can't eat – and the establishment of a set of rules around food and eating simplifies the world by coming up with simple answers, in the same way that religions set out simple rules for living (e.g. 'Thou shalt not kill'). Food cults and diets therefore ease the stress of navigating the huge abundance of choices and conflicting information we're faced with daily, by providing us with rules and norms, with pseudoscientific reasoning that gives the simple nutritional answers we desire.

Food cults utilise all the tricks of the trade. Evidence is shunned in favour of anecdotes and testimonials from converts, endorsement from authority or celebrity figures, group validation and the sharing of a common enemy. Although scientific thinking can be used to combat pseudoscience, it takes practice and effort, and food science is particularly complex and rife with misinformation. After all, 'The amount of energy necessary to refute bullshit is an order of magnitude bigger than to produce it' – so said Italian programmer Alberto Brandolini. We have a modern food environment with almost limitless choice and convenience, which is the ideal setting for the promotion of food cults and diets that make this choice easier for us. Unfortunately, most people do not have the skills necessary to navigate the information and misinformation relating to diet and nutrition encountered on a daily basis, and it's something we just aren't taught unless we do a science degree – and even then, it's not a guarantee. Add the Internet and social media to that and you have misinformation spreading like wildfire. Pseudoscientific nutrition claims and food cults have a ubiquitous presence in society, and these food cults are most likely here to stay. But by being aware of them, recognising the harm they can do and trying our best to counter any misinformation, we can at least make a start.

'You are what you eat' is a popular notion, and as I mentioned above, it kind of makes sense to us. The belief that we absorb and transfer the physical and moral qualities of the food we eat is near universal. Religious studies professor Alan Levinovitz shares a number of examples of these in his book, *The Gluten Lie*:

> Native Americans believed that eating venison made you fleet of foot, while eating clumsy bears, helpless dung-hill fowls, and the 'heavy wallowing swine' made you slower, both physically and mentally. In Turkey, children slow to speak were fed bird tongues. Traditional Zulu doctors prescribed the ground bones of old cows so their patients might absorb longevity. To jump higher, Northern Australian aborigines ate kangaroo and emu. The Mishing people of India fed tiger to men as a means of fortifying their strength, but not to women.

So much of traditional Chinese medicine is based on this concept, but is thankfully fading now that the ivory trade is illegal and there was worldwide outrage over the killing of animals such as tigers and rhinoceroses. That superstition that you are what you eat is still pervasive today, particularly in the narrative that 'if you eat fat you will become fat', or more simply 'fat makes you fat'. This has since sparked a whole bunch of counter-articles that claim 'fat doesn't make you fat' (because carbs apparently do) (they don't).

Historically, dietary reformists like Sylvester Graham, creator of the graham cracker (similar to the digestive biscuit in the UK), took this a step further by connecting the logic of 'You are what you eat' to morals. Graham was a clergyman who practised vegetarianism, and strongly believed that eating animal meat would exacerbate animal instinct, which is why people were craving food and sex and becoming fat and promiscuous. He collected anecdotes, and, just like the paleo crowd of today, he used evolutionary biology to justify his stance. But where the paleo group claim that we should eat like hunter-gatherers because that's what we are designed to do, Graham said that because humans don't have sharp teeth like carnivores, we therefore shouldn't eat meat. And so it no longer became an argument about health alone: it was also about human virtue and having a strong moral stance.

Interestingly, with sugar the historical argument was similar to vegetarianism. There it was argued that because sugar was produced and imported in immoral ways (namely slavery), it would have negative consequences on your body. You eat something immoral and it will manifest in your body, because it makes you an immoral person. We even see an example of this in popular culture, where evil characters eat questionable things and are ugly because their evil manifests itself in the form of physical ugliness; whereas the good protagonists are attractive because their virtue manifests itself in the form of physical beauty.

Dieting has been incredibly feminised throughout history, as apparently 'real men don't diet'. Food-related activities, such as shopping, cooking and eating, are conventionally presented as female-centred and part of the female identity, while men are the clueless recipients of food. But more recently cultural pressures have been bearing down on men too, which has resulted in the popularity of the ketogenic diet and paleo movement. These movements make dieting manly again by masculinising 'You are what you eat' – if you eat meat you will become strong and muscly and manly, how men are supposed to be. But it isn't seen as a diet so much as a way of life, as both tend to be accompanied by strict exercise regimes. If the goal is weight loss, then exercise is seen as the way to achieve that, whereas eating meat is for building muscle. Paleo makes men think back to a time where they were strong cavemen who cared for the family by hunting animals, a time long before feminine diets, which makes it more palatable. The idea of eating muscle (meat) to gain muscle has long been a popular one; I'm sure we've all heard the phrases 'beef up' and 'strong as an ox'. Since the ideal body shape for men is portrayed as being lean and muscular, it's no wonder that lean meat is the food of choice to obtain this.

We have focused so much on the simple phrase 'You are what you eat' that it puts the emphasis on you as a person: if you are fat and sick it must be your fault, because you choose what you eat. Is it any wonder that fat people are stereotyped as being lazy, weak-willed, greedy and unattractive? Compare this with serious cases of anorexia, where people are not blamed, or told to get their act together, or seen as weak. No, they're seen as having amazing willpower, and are even praised by some individuals. But it's not their fault. The inconsistency is incredible.

Diet culture lies to us about health

Diet culture bombards us with messages about the value of our health and bodies everywhere we go. Products, services, diets, gyms, pills – all this information overwhelms us. We can't escape the messages of dieting and weight loss. Two-thirds of us are on a diet most of the time.

So where has all this dieting got us? Not far. We are a population terrified of being fat, and yet many of us *are* fat. This fear of fatness has made us endlessly restrict our food, have our jaws clamped shut, have our stomachs stapled, start smoking, do crazy exercise routines, and hate ourselves.

People have an increasingly problematic relationship with food, and we can thank a variety of factors for this. First, beauty ideals have shifted over the last few decades, and the curvaceous symbol of fertility has now shifted into a thin, slender body. Second, this body ideal has merged with a diet culture that has fat bodies as the enemy. Third is the rise of 'healthism', where health becomes a moral imperative and health is purely the responsibility of the individual. So social constructions of health have captured public attention and placed responsibility on the individual to prevent ill health; and at the same time they have linked moral obligation and worthiness to the size and shape of bodies.

It's now normal for people to be dissatisfied with their bodies. It's so rare to find someone without body hang-ups that you'd be forgiven for thinking such people don't exist (or are narcissists). Estimates vary, but generally around 70 per cent to over 90 per cent of women, and over half of men, are dissatisfied with their bodies. This develops early in life, in children as young as seven years old, and isn't limited to a single body size, ethnicity, sexual orientation or identity. Research has identified body dissatisfaction as one of the most consistent and robust risk factors for eating disorders, low self-esteem and depression. So, in many ways, body dissatisfaction has emerged as a core aspect of our physical and mental health. Why is it that so many people are dissatisfied with their bodies, regardless of their size? Although parental influences and bullying play a role, there has been a huge rise in portrayal of the ideal body shape in the media. This ideal body is thin for women, and lean and muscular for men. Across all forms of media and social media, the thin and lean ideals are constantly emphasised, rewarded and praised, while fat characters are either the funny friend, the 'before' photo, or depicted as unlovable. The women illustrated in the media today are becoming thinner and thinner, and are far smaller than the average woman who receives these images. Similarly, the men illustrated have become more and more muscular over time. Both these images portray something that is unrealistic for most of the population.

Exposure to television commercials that feature the thin-ideal image (as opposed to average-weight women or images that aren't appearance-related) increases women's body dissatisfaction while images of muscular men make the average man feel small and inadequate. But advertisers take advantage of this and use it to sell us things we don't need, to fix problems we didn't even have to begin with. Diet culture loves this, because it can make mountains of money off our insecurities and our vulnerabilities.

Diet culture has lied to us about our health in so many ways. It tells us that we can only be healthy if we are thin, that hunger is bad, that eating when you are sad is wrong, that there are 'good' and 'bad' foods, that we must exercise to lose weight, and that our bodies aren't good enough. It broadcasts this around the world for us to see on our TV screens and on our social media apps. Diet culture tells us that our bodies dictate our worth, and that it is our fault if we are unhealthy.

Diet culture is wrong.

Throughout this book, I want to tackle the various lies we've been told about our health and nutrition, and how believing these lies has had the opposite effect to what we expect: it's made us unhealthier than before. And it's made us fall out of love with food. Food is no longer something to be celebrated; for many people, food is a daily source of anxiety, and something to do battle with.

Yes, I'm a nutritionist, and it's my job to help people live healthier lives, but what I'm seeing in clinic saddens and worries me. Nutrition is important, of course it is, but it's become exaggerated and distorted. Even the term 'good food', which was once reserved for tables piled high with delicious dishes, now suggests something entirely different. Now good food is not about the pleasure of eating but is concerned with the good health that results from our dietary choices.

Nutrition did not invent a morality about eating, even if it rehearses it. Nutrition merely mapped on to existing concerns about food and pleasure. Food is supposed to be pleasurable; it's wired into our very DNA. Food is so much more than just the nutrients it gives us to survive, and health is so much more than just the food we eat. It's time we reminded ourselves of that, and took back the pleasure that diet culture robbed us of.

References

Contois, E.J. (2015). 'Guilt-free and sinfully delicious: a contemporary theology of weight loss dieting'. *Fat Studies*, 4(2):112–26.

Rozin, P. (1996). 'Towards a psychology of food and eating: From motivation to module to model to marker, morality, meaning, and metaphor'. *Current Directions in Psychological Science*, 5(1):18–24.

Levinovitz, A. (2015). *The Gluten Lie: and other myths about what you eat.* Simon and Schuster.

Gough, B. (2007). '"Real men don't diet": An analysis of contemporary newspaper representations of men, food and health'. *Social Science & Medicine*, 64(2):326–37.

2

WEIGHT AND HEALTH

*'Insanity is doing the same thing over and over again
and expecting different results.'*

NOT ALBERT EINSTEIN*

The public health 'war on obesity' has, let's face it, not exactly been successful. Despite the nation going on diet after diet, obesity levels have continued to rise. Why is this?

The campaigns to prevent and tackle obesity have placed a huge focus on individual responsibility. Surely it makes sense to focus on weight if you're trying to get people to not be obese? Well, no, not quite. This is what we've been led to believe. But it's a bit more complicated than that.

It seems simple: if you're overweight, it means you're unhealthy, and you need to go on a diet to lose weight. This is the dogma of our society and it is so ingrained that we don't question it. Well, I say it's time to question it. This dogma has a name, and it's known as the 'weight-normative approach'.

* Although this quote is always attributed to Albert Einstein, there is no record of him saying this and it has been thoroughly debunked. But there's no denying it's a great quote.

The main assumptions of the weight-normative approach are:

1. Excess weight causes disease and early death.
2. Weight loss is required for better health and is the best treatment option.
3. Focusing on weight and weight loss is not harmful.

Despite the fact that the weight-normative approach is everywhere and accepted as the norm, from health to healthcare to diet conversations between friends, the overall evidence doesn't support this approach. It's neither effective nor ethical. Let's examine each of these assumptions and the overwhelming evidence that should force us to completely rethink how much we equate weight with health.

1) Excess weight causes disease and early death.

The assumption here is that the higher your weight, the more at risk you are of developing various diseases and the more likely you are to die prematurely. But it goes even beyond that, suggesting that excess weight is the cause of disease and the cause of death.

We measure weight in research not because it accurately reflects health but simply because it is really easy to measure. No invasive blood tests or special equipment required, which also allows for the easy tracking of changes over time. Add height to this and we have the most commonly used tool to assess health: Body Mass Index, or BMI.

$$BMI = \text{weight in kg} / \text{height in m squared}$$

A quick reminder of BMI categories:

- 'Underweight' BMI <18.5
- 'Normal' BMI 18.5–25
- 'Overweight' BMI 25–30
- 'Obese' BMI 30–35
- 'Morbidly obese' BMI >35

BMI has many issues. It's useful and interesting when assessing the health of a large-scale population but was never intended to be used on individuals. Not all body weight is equal, but BMI assumes it is. The example of rugby players is often used, as they tend to have large amounts of muscle, which puts them firmly in the 'overweight' BMI category even if they don't have high body fat. It's a simple example of the shortcomings of BMI that many accept; however, few would argue that these people are unhealthy. What about instances where someone is in the 'overweight' BMI category due to fat tissue rather than muscle tissue? Even then it's not simple, as location of fat also matters. A large accumulation of fat cells in the central trunk is more harmful than body fat in other places. Also known as visceral fat, it gathers around the body's organs, as opposed to subcutaneous fat, which sits under the skin.

Increased BMI may be linked to various diseases, I don't deny that, but causation often cannot be established, and there are a whole host of confounding variables that often don't get corrected for in research. These include other lifestyle factors such as exercise, nutrition and stress, as well as socio-economic and genetic factors. We cannot categorically say that excess weight *causes* a lot of disease.

When it comes to mortality, that's where things get interesting. The assumption would be that 'obese' people are more likely to die prematurely than those in the 'overweight' category, and these are more likely to die prematurely than those in the 'normal' category. However, that just isn't the case.

Risk of dying prematurely is highest among both the 'underweight' and 'morbidly obese' categories, and lowest among both the 'normal' and 'overweight' categories. That's right, being 'overweight' doesn't mean you're more likely to die prematurely than being at a 'normal' weight.[1] In fact, after analysing almost three million adults worldwide, the conclusion was that being 'overweight' actually decreases your risk of early death relative to 'normal' weight. Is your mind blown? It should be.

The 'obesity paradox' is so-called because obesity is associated with better survival in diseases such as type 2 diabetes, hypertension and heart disease. Overweight elderly people also live longer than their thin counterparts.[2]

Many factors influence health, and body weight is just one small part of it. Determining a person's health by their weight is like trying to describe the complete picture of a puzzle when you only have one piece.

2) Weight loss is required for better health and is the best treatment option.

The diet industry consists of books, DVDs, magazines, supplements, special foods, subscription programmes and more. If I ask you to think of a diet, what comes to mind? Something like Weight Watchers or Slimming World, or the Cabbage Soup diet?

A diet is arguably any form of eating that has a set of rules that can be broken. Anything with a list of foods you have to avoid is a diet. A diet tells you when to eat, what to eat and how much to eat. If you have rules, if you can 'mess up', if you have to follow a plan or if you have to count or track anything, then it's a diet. It might not like to admit it's a diet, it might call itself a lifestyle instead (like 'clean eating' or paleo), but that doesn't stop it from being a diet.

The diet industry relies on framing weight gain as a personal responsibility by providing solutions in the form of weight loss products and programmes.

At the time of writing, the global diet industry was calculated to be worth $168.95 billion: $70.3 billion of that is from the US (almost $1.5 billion from WeightWatchers alone) and over £2 billion from the UK.

The entire business model of the diet industry is based around diets failing. The industry has a huge amount to gain from it – weight-loss failures mean repeat customers and more profit. It sounds cynical, but it makes sense when you think about it: if there was a diet that was completely successful, everyone would do it and would succeed, and that would be the end of that. But that's not what happens. Instead, you do the 12-week programme (or however many weeks they tell you), lose a little (or a lot) of weight at the beginning, struggle to maintain that, give up because you can't maintain the set of rules you have to follow, and end up back where you started. You're demoralised, ashamed, and on top of that, you're made to feel like it's all YOUR fault.

Right now, you're probably thinking 'But I know some-one /read about someone / I myself have followed X plan and managed to lose X amount of weight and keep it off'! Well, good for you. But that's an anecdote, and just because you know someone for whom something has worked doesn't make it a raging success. It takes more than a few anecdotes for us to be able to conclude that something 'works'. If a drug worked for you but had an 80 per cent failure rate, would you call it successful on a population level? No. Well, believe it or not, that's the failure rate of diets.

Looking at the statistics, it makes you wonder why people bother with diets at all:

* Although many interventions generate weight loss in the short term, the research shows that less than 20 per cent maintain weight loss after one year,[3] and even less after two years. I think it's important to note that those 20 per cent only maintained their weight loss by weighing themselves regularly, doing around an hour of exercise PER DAY, and eating a carefully monitored low-calorie diet that didn't allow for wiggle room at the weekends. Doesn't that sound enjoyable?
* Of those who had maintained their weight loss, around a quarter said they felt highly stressed, depressed, and dissatisfied with their weight loss.
* The Women's Health Initiative in the US (the largest and longest trial on weight loss) found that after seven and a half years, the more than 20,000 women did not, on average, have a different weight compared with the start.[4]
* Experts have determined that 'one-third to two-thirds of the weight is regained within one year, and almost all is regained within five years'.[5]
* Beyond simply unsuccessfully losing weight, one-third to two-thirds of dieters end up regaining more weight than they lost on their diets, so end up heavier than before.[6]

- After two years, individuals who report trying to diet end up a higher weight than before.[7]
- Children whose parents put them on diets and restrict food intake are more likely to eat even when not hungry and be overweight later in life.[8]

In all likelihood, the real-world statistics are even less encouraging than studies show. Weight-loss studies often have high drop-out rates (people are more likely to drop out if they feel the diet isn't working or they can't follow it) and those who drop out aren't included in the final analysis, meaning a great many people for whom the diet failed aren't taken into account at the end of a study. Naturally, this makes the diet look more successful, as the participants left at the end tend to be the most successful dieters and inflate the results. Participants in weight-loss studies also tend to have far more contact with healthcare professionals than the average person trying to lose weight at home. Seeing a dietitian every few weeks is a far bigger motivator, as well as them being someone participants can turn to for guidance and to answer questions. Most people who embark on a diet try something at home or pay to join a commercial weight-loss programme. Very few of these programmes publish their results and tend to stick to individual anecdotes instead, but the limited research we do have suggests that the largest weight loss was around 3.2 per cent of body weight after two years.[9] Are you underwhelmed? 'Cause I sure am.

On top of all that, you have to consider publication bias – scientific journals are far more likely to publish a study that shows a significant effect over something that didn't work.

Weight-loss programmes in the workplace and in schools

have been equally unsuccessful. Despite appearing to be very concerned about the students' growing waistlines, very few schools actually assess the impact of making nutritional changes on pupils' weight. When they do, the results aren't exactly promising either, as simple techniques like discouraging fizzy drinks have pretty much no effect at all.[10] The lack of research in this area allows people to continue to think that school interventions are successful, as there is no published evidence to the contrary. Yet we hear reports about 'childhood obesity constantly rising'.

Similarly, in the workplace the average weight loss among people who take part in these programmes is 3 lb (1.36 kg) more than those who don't join in.[11] That's after a year of taking part. After four years, there's no difference between the two groups at all. Again, incredibly underwhelming.

When researchers investigated the impact of weight loss on health and mortality, they concluded that weight loss in healthy obese individuals increased risk of mortality rather than decreased it, as would be expected. They suggested that weight loss should only be advised for those with obesity-related diseases such as type 2 diabetes.[12] At this point, though, I think it's worth mentioning that there is more to this picture than simple risk of dying, and there is more to health than just type 2 diabetes and heart disease. Looking at the population as a whole (UK, US, EU, or Australian, for example), these are definitely incredibly significant contributors to health and mortality, but it doesn't take into account more minor factors like osteoarthritis and sleep apnoea (both are known to be related to body weight), which may not kill but can still disrupt a person's well-being.

A detailed analysis of the scientific literature used to justify weight-management initiatives as a matter of public health came to the conclusion that 'dietetic literature on weight management fails to meet the standards of evidence-based medicine'.[13] A damning statement indeed. Researchers were found to exaggerate conclusions made in referenced studies, and reference in loops that went round and round without actually citing an original source. The assumption that weight loss is a good thing is so ingrained that researchers don't even feel the need to justify why they were seeking this outcome. In scientific research you normally have to justify *everything*. So why is weight loss exempt from this?

Short-term weight-loss intervention studies (up to six months) usually find improvements in health measures such as cholesterol or blood pressure. But we cannot tell if these short-term outcomes are due to the weight loss itself or due to the behaviour changes. This may not sound significant, but it is important to disentangle the two to understand exactly what is beneficial here. This is really difficult to do, though. We do have one good example: liposuction. Liposuction is an example of weight loss without behaviour change, and although significant weight is lost (I mean, it's literally sucked out of the body), afterwards there are generally no improvements in health measures such as blood pressure, triglycerides or cholesterol. So, when we have weight loss without behaviour change, we don't see metabolic improvements. Looking at studies on type 2 diabetes, improvements in blood-sugar control is seen within a few days, long before anyone has the chance to lose any significant weight. This suggests that the behaviour change is what's having a positive effect on their overall health.

The other important question we need to ask ourselves is why diets work in the short term but not in the long term. Essentially: why do diets fail? Can we ascribe this 80-per-cent failure rate simply to lack of willpower? Hell, no.

You may be surprised to know that your body doesn't necessarily want you to lose weight. There are strong biological systems in place that respond to a reduced energy intake by lowering your metabolism, increasing your levels of hunger, increasing food-related thoughts and making food seem more desirable and appealing. Essentially, by dieting you are fighting your body and your own biology every step of the way.

There is evidence that there is a biological control of body weight at any given point, and each one of us has a 'set point' at which our bodies comfortably sit.[14] This set point is the result of our genetics and our environment. When we try to deviate from this set point, our body adjusts things like metabolism, food intake and energy expenditure in order to maintain and defend this set point. Your set point isn't going to be an exact number but a fairly narrow range of weight that your body is happy with. The question on your lips right now is probably: 'So why is it so easy to gain weight but hard to lose it again?' Increasing the amount of energy you use (mainly through movement) will trigger an increase in appetite to make up for that extra energy spent, resulting in an energy balance. But the reverse isn't true; if you increase your energy intake, you won't automatically feel the need to move more and expend more energy. It seems that set point is asymmetrical, which explains why it's so easy to regain lost weight, but so hard to lose gained weight. The body seems to defend against weight loss far more effectively than against weight gain. From an evolutionary perspective, this does make some sense: preventing our body losing weight is a protective mechanism to ensure we don't starve in times of food scarcity, whereas in times of food abundance we (historically) would want to eat as much as possible and store that weight for harsher times. But, of course, our environment has drastically changed and we are now lucky enough to live in a society where food scarcity is much rarer; instead we have constant food abundance. This imperfect body control is now at odds with our present lifestyle, but this still doesn't make weight gain our fault – it still derives from external factors. When we eat a healthy balanced diet without restriction and with some movement, we tend to stay around our set point. But when we diet, this biological mechanism steps into gear and can remain active for a year afterwards.[14] The theory is by no means perfect, as it doesn't take into account a whole myriad of other factors that affect human behaviour, but I find whenever I explain this concept to clients it makes so much sense for them.

Going on a diet generally involves rules that have the explicit intention of putting you into a calorie deficit, which means your energy intake will be lower than your energy expenditure and you'll lose weight. With any kind of energy deficit, but especially the kind where you're expected to live off 800–1,200 kcals (calories) a day, you're eating less than what your body needs for basic functioning, and your body doesn't like that. Your body understandably can't tell the difference between genuine unplanned starvation and a strict diet (voluntary starvation, if you prefer). Your body doesn't have that level of insight. So the response is the same: decrease metabolism and increase hunger hormones. There are two main possible outcomes: either you ignore your increased hunger (as often seen in cases of anorexia nervosa) and your body eventually gives up and shuts your hunger hormones off to save energy; or you are unable to fight these powerful signals, in which case you end up overeating – cue feelings of guilt and shame for not being able to stick to your diet. Even if someone does manage to ignore their biological signals and suppress their weight and maintain it, the dietary rigidity needed to achieve that increases the risk of eating disorders, particularly bulimia, due to the almost inevitable binge that follows restriction. The research (and I'm sure your own personal experience) backs this up: rigid dieting is usually broken up by episodes of overeating, even in the absence of hunger.[15] You diet and restrict, then you overeat, you beat yourself up about it, and you diet again. And so the cycle goes on.

As I mentioned, weight loss leads to a reduction in metabolic rate, which makes it harder to maintain the suppressed weight. So a person with a certain BMI who has never dieted would be able to eat more kcals than someone who had dieted down to that BMI and still maintain that weight.[16]

It's important to remember that these metabolic and hormonal changes can stick around for a good year after weight loss. Increased hunger and hunger hormones are common a full year later, while fullness hormones are decreased.[17] This matches the reduced metabolic rate after weight loss and it has been suggested that this helps explain why most people end up regaining the weight they lost.

The sense of failure when weight loss is unsuccessful places the blame squarely on the individual. We say, 'I've failed', 'I've fallen off the wagon', 'I need to get back on track'. But should we really be blaming the individuals when the concept of the diet itself is what's at fault?

Beyond trying to fight our own biology, there is a whole host of other factors that affect our weight, such as our food environment, genetics, socio-economic factors, how much income you have available for food, how much time you have to prepare food, what equipment you have available, what cooking skills you do or don't have, medication, psychological factors – the list goes on. Overall, there are huge limitations on the degree to which body weight can voluntarily be altered. Placing the emphasis on 'healthy weight' as the key can lead people to feel hopeless when their efforts are unsuccessful. This can lead people to think that making positive lifestyle changes is pointless. Which it absolutely is not.

Permanent weight loss is not the norm for most people on a diet. But people can benefit and become healthier from lifestyle interventions even if their weight remains stable. The current available research supports this. Lifestyle changes can improve blood pressure, blood lipids and insulin sensitivity completely independently of weight.[18]

When researchers examined the effects of following four health-promoting behaviours on overall mortality in the UK, those who engaged in all four – non-smoking, physically active, moderate alcohol intake and five servings of fruit and vegetables a day – had a hugely reduced risk of early death, equivalent to living 14 years longer than someone who engages in none of these behaviours. This effect was independent of BMI.[19]

Similarly, in the US, when people engaged in all four of these health-promoting behaviours, the risk of mortality was equal across the BMI spectrum.[20] The findings reinforced the relationship between healthy lifestyle habits and decreased risk of death independent of BMI. This is hugely important, as it shows that health-promoting behaviours improve health for everyone (not just those in larger bodies) and really provides a good rationale for promoting health over weight. Sure, for some people, engaging in these behaviours may result in weight loss, while for others it may not, but that doesn't negate the benefits these behaviours provide and so should be taken seriously. Similarly, those at a lower BMI may believe that following these healthy behaviours isn't as important because of their 'healthy' weight, when in fact their health would still be significantly improved.

Collectively, these studies sampled almost 100,000 people. That's a lot of people.

So why do the vast majority of people, including healthcare professionals, push the narrative that weight loss is the goal, and that it's attainable? The research about weight loss being unsuccessful long term has been replicated many times; it's been published in prestigious journals and communicated in the media to the public. Why are we not listening?

People like simple arguments and simple solutions. Many healthcare professionals are invested in weight management as a part of their practice, and work in settings where promoting the notion of 'eat less, move more, it's simple' is the norm.[21] This message sounds so compelling, even though it's not true – if it were really that simple, there wouldn't be any fat people. In addition, weight loss and dieting is big business, and if weight loss were simple, then this industry wouldn't exist because it wouldn't be needed. But it is such a huge industry, and we see weight-loss advertisements everywhere we go, with testimonials from the handful of people who have had success (or those who had success after 12 weeks before regaining all the weight again after, but you don't put that part on a billboard). Weight-loss programmes make hugely unrealistic bold claims, which we internalise and believe, because we want to believe. The 'before' and 'after' photos that are so pervasive in weight-loss advertising, that are such a big part of the personal transformation – glorify the future and the possibilities that will be available then, at the expense of the past and present.[22] This encourages people to put their life on hold for the sake of the future, and creates the illusion that progress is inevitable, and that success is just around the corner.

Of course we want to believe it's possible, because in our society a fat body is a bad body, whereas a thin body is a good body. The weight-normative approach promotes the view that people of higher weights are unhealthy and a financial burden on society, and that weight is under the control of the individual; therefore if someone is fat, then it's because they're not trying to be healthier. I think, based on the evidence available, we can agree that this is a gross oversimplification of health.

The Foresight obesity model* includes over 100 drivers of obesity and over 300 interconnections acting in complex feedback loops. Put into this context, is it really surprising that government campaigns are overly simplistic and therefore unlikely to work? I don't think so. Focusing purely on responsibility of the individual paves the way for blaming or punishing those whose choices are deemed unhealthy or not good enough.

---

*   The Foresight obesity model is a map which looks at all the factors that can affect body weight, ranging from biological and medical to food and psychological factors.

We blame the individual, and this has unintended consequences, as we're about to find out.

3) Focusing on weight and weight loss is not harmful.

I've already touched on some of the negative psychological impacts dieting can have, such as lower self-esteem and body-image issues. Placing body shape and size as being of the utmost importance can encourage people to use any means necessary to achieve that 'ideal', 'healthy' weight, even relying on behaviours more commonly associated with eating disorders, such as purging and fasting. But these behaviours are hidden, and people will likely be praised for 'trying to be healthier' even if their methods are far from it. However the potential negative effects of weight loss go far beyond that.

A weight-focused approach may lead to both 'false negatives' (a misdiagnosis as healthy due to 'normal' weight) as well as 'false positives' (misdiagnosing larger patients as unhealthy and prescribing weight loss). Both of these carry potential risks for people across the BMI spectrum.

There are several known physiological side effects of dieting. For one, reduced bone mass, which increases the risk of osteoporosis. Individuals on a calorie-restricted diet are less likely to be getting all the nutrients they need, including those important for bone health such as calcium. Dieting also increases chronic stress and cortisol production (the stress hormone), which increases disease risk. Finally, we know that dieting is a strong predictor of future weight gain.[2]

Dieting failure is often accompanied by weight cycling, more commonly known as yo-yo dieting – where weight regularly cycles up and down and up and down. Research has shown a link between weight cycling and several negative health outcomes such as higher risk of early death, loss of muscle, high blood pressure, chronic inflammation, heart disease, stroke, diabetes and some types of cancer.[23-25] Most significantly, weight cycling is linked to negative psychological outcomes such as depression, anxiety, less physical activity, more binge-eating and lower self-esteem.

Across the world, people in larger bodies are stereotyped as lazy, lacking willpower, incompetent, unattractive, and to blame for their weight. I think almost all of us can put our hands up and say we've thought some of these thoughts when we see a fat person, particularly a fat person eating in public. When it comes to dieting and the weight-focused approach, the biggest and most unappreciated side effect is weight stigma.

Weight stigma includes weight-related teasing, bullying, harassment, violence, hostility, ostracism, pressure to lose weight, and microaggressions such as being asked to purchase two plane tickets instead of one. Weight discrimination has increased over the years to a similar level to that of race and age discrimination.[26]

Weight bias is an example of social inequity, as people in larger bodies are treated differently from those in smaller bodies. It occurs on public transport, in healthcare, employment, education and so on. This is an example of what is known as 'thin privilege'. Someone in a smaller body may experience the same internal dissatisfaction with their body as someone in a larger body, but they are far less likely to be subjected to the same prejudice by society. That is the key difference.

One particular example is in a healthcare setting. Patients in larger bodies are typically evaluated first based on their weight, regardless of whether it is relevant to the problem they've presented with. When weight loss is made the number-one priority, it affects how healthcare professionals think about weight and health. Weight bias has been documented in dietitians, doctors, nurses and psychologists. For example, psychologists will say that a fat patient has more severe symptoms and a worse prognosis compared with when a patient is thin, even if they present with identical psychological profiles.[27] Of particular note, an assessment of trainee dietitians, doctors, nurses and nutritionists showed that 98 per cent had some degree of fatphobia and negative attitudes towards people in larger bodies.[28] These are the future healthcare professionals who are supposed to be treating us for any health issues we may face. This bias is completely unacceptable, as experiencing weight bias from healthcare professionals may discourage patients from seeking help or guidance, particularly for problems unrelated to weight.

Medical professionals prescribing weight loss and seeking 'healthy weight' encourages societal messages that say there is only one acceptable and ideal aesthetic: thinness for women and leanness for men. Internalisation of these ideals is related to shame, body dissatisfaction, eating disorders, body dysmorphia and muscle dysmorphia.[29,30] Let's not forget that obesity and eating disorders are not mutually exclusive. They can, and do, coexist, and they have risk factors in common.

Those who experience high levels of weight bias internalisation are significantly more likely to have metabolic syndrome – a collection of conditions such as high blood pressure and abnormal cholesterol levels.[31] Individuals with metabolic syndrome have a 2x increased risk for heart disease and a 5x increased risk for type 2 diabetes.[32] It is possible that as those with metabolic syndrome often experience stigma by health-care professionals, the increased need for healthcare may increase the exposure to stigma and so increase the likelihood of internalising it. So it may actually be a reverse association. Hard to tell. Either way, it's a problem.

Weight stigma is a chronic stressor and elicits a stress response in the body. This increases blood pressure and cortisol reactivity, leading to increased appetite and binge-eating. Weight stigma is associated with increased risk for depression, anxiety, body dissatisfaction and low self-esteem. Perceived weight stigma increases the risk of dying prematurely by over 50 per cent.[33]

Weight stigma has repeatedly been shown to be a separate and unique factor affecting health outcomes and health behaviours. Both adults and children who experience weight stigma are less likely to engage in healthful behaviours like physical activity and eating a healthy, balanced diet. Weight stigma reduces quality of life and interferes with people's well-meaning attempts to lose weight and improve their health, often leading to weight gain instead.[34]

Adolescents who experience teasing about their weight show higher levels of unhealthy food behaviours such as fasting, purging or binge-eating.[35] This is true for both boys and girls, and whether those comments come from family or friends. Among adults, research consistently shows a link between stigma and eating behaviours such as dieting, binge-eating, emotional eating and even eating disorders.[36] In weight-loss camps in particular, stigma is associated with binge-eating and more extreme weight-control behaviours like fasting and purging. In general, the more experiences with weight stigma a person has on a particular day, the less motivated they are to diet and to lose weight. Experiences with weight stigma in people's everyday lives can negatively impact their motivation and eating behaviour.

The behavioural consequences of weight stigma matter just as much as the physiological consequences because they have the opposite effect than intended: people are less likely to lose weight and more likely to gain weight over time.[36]

In addition, the stigma associated with weight may actually be causing some of the negative health outcomes associated with a higher weight, rather than the weight itself.

The very term 'lifestyle diseases', which includes obesity, is not entirely accurate as there is a whole host of other factors besides lifestyle that are known to affect them. Factors such as genetics and environmental influences are well outside personal control. The groups of people with the worst health outcomes are also those at the lower end of the socio-economic scale, who have the least control over their lives and their lifestyle.[37] Despite this, current public health messaging focuses too much on factors that are more within our personal control, and overlooks the larger sociocultural and economic conditions that dictate much of people's lived experiences, choices and opportunities.

It's not only weight stigma between individuals that has harmful effects, but also weight-focused public health policies. Policies that place the focus on weight are based on limited evidence and ignore the root cause of issues, focusing instead on the outcomes of weight. They teach the public that weight needs to be our focus, and these policies can lead to body dissatisfaction, disordered eating, discrimination and even death from eating disorders, surgery complications, or suicide as a result of bullying.[38]

The literature suggests that the word 'obese' is more stigmatising to people in larger bodies than 'fat', and because of that you'll find me using the word 'fat' or 'person in a larger body' wherever possible in the rest of this book. I refuse to use language that over-medicalises people's bodies and makes them feel unnecessarily bad about themselves. The National Institute for Health and Care Excellence (NICE) guidelines* overlook this, despite telling healthcare professionals to be careful with their terminology.[39] When shown obesity-related public health campaigns, people responded less favourably to messages that were stigmatising, and showed less inclination to comply with the messages. However, messages that focused on healthy behaviours without mentioning the word 'obesity' were much more positively received and motivating.[40]

I don't claim to be a public health expert, but clearly we need to rethink the strategies by which we bring health messages to the population. If the evidence clearly shows that the way we currently do things (i.e. focusing on weight and weight loss) doesn't work, then we need to shift our focus to health gain and healthful behaviours. Public health messages should focus on health and well-being for all, not simply weight reduction for some.

As we have already seen, following four simple health-promoting behaviours decreases mortality for *everyone*, regardless of their BMI.[20] If public health messaging focused on health-promoting behaviours in a non-discriminatory way, encouraging people of all shapes and sizes to follow them, the implications

* NICE is an independent public body that provides national guidance and advice to improve health and social care in England, with some services to Wales, Scotland and Northern Ireland.

would be far more effective and far-reaching than stigmatising and unhelpful campaigns such as 'Obesity causes cancer', which is neither accurate (there is an association but not causation) nor helpful in terms of changing behaviour.

Interventions to prevent weight bias could include legislation to prohibit weight discrimination, showing positive experiences of people in larger bodies in the media (rather than just the 'funny one' or making weight loss the entire basis of their character development), or offering school programmes geared towards positive body image, body diversity, and awareness and prevention of weight biases.

Overall, we just can't justify using weight bias as a public health tactic to address 'the obesity epidemic'. All people, regardless of body size, deserve respect, equity and dignity, and to live without stigma and discrimination. We have made leaps and bounds in achieving this when it comes to homophobia and discrimination based on sexuality; now it's time to extend that to weight. We don't say that the way to eradicate homophobia is to remove all LGBTQ+ folks, and we can't say that in order to remove weight stigma we have to just remove all higher weight people.

When it comes to weight stigma, fat women experience far worse discrimination than men do, whether it's in the workplace, in romantic relationships, in education settings or in healthcare.[41] Overall, fat women are less likely to be hired, receive worse treatment while doing their job, and earn less than their thin peers. Fat women are less likely to be married, whereas fat men are not. Fat black women have an even worse time of it. This intersectionality of racism, misogynism and weight stigma is significant, as much of the research on weight stigma has focused on white women, but black women experience proportionately more weight-based discrimination. This dismisses and invalidates the experiences fat black women go through, and the increased stress they are under as a result. Fat bodies are already seen as less valuable in society, and fat black bodies even more so, because the ideal standard of beauty is still thin and white.

Let's be honest, if shame were an effective motivator for weight loss, there wouldn't be many fat people around. As it is, we KNOW it doesn't work. In fact, we know it's likely to have the opposite effect to the one intended, with additional negative psychological side effects. We have known this for a while; it isn't anything new. Yet we want to believe that shame works, because it's easier to continue to be disgusted by fat people or claim that we're being cruel because we care about their health, rather than just admitting the truth: we're prejudiced against a group of people purely for the way they look. 'I'm not racist but...', 'I'm not homophobic but...', 'I'm not fatphobic but...'. Racism, homophobia, fatphobia. All prejudices based on someone's appearance. Fatphobia is just still more socially acceptable.

If people who fat-shame others really were doing it out of a concern for their health, they'd also be focusing their attentions on thin people who smoke, or people who regularly take drugs. Or what about people who are underweight or malnourished? The most recent estimated cost of malnutrition in England at the time of writing was £19.6 billion, affecting three million people in the UK. In comparison, the most recent estimated cost of obesity in the UK was £6.1 billion, with projected costs of £9.7 billion by 2050 – which is still considerably lower than the cost of malnutrition. Fat-shaming really has nothing to do with worrying about someone's health. It's making an assumption about someone's health based on their appearance, simply because you don't like the way they look.

It's not all doom and gloom: enter the weight-inclusive approach

The weight-normative approach puts weight loss as the primary goal despite extensive evidence that weight loss isn't sustainable in the long term for most people,[3,7,18] that weight cycling is linked to adverse effects,[23-25] and that the stigma this perpetuates does even greater harm.

Enter the alternative way of thinking: the weight-inclusive approach. This approach rests on the assumption that everyone is capable of achieving health and well-being independent of weight, if they are not discriminated against and are given access to non-stigmatising healthcare. Here weight is not the primary focus of medical treatment or health intervention.

This approach tries to minimise weight stigma, so the blame for being unable to lose weight is placed on the process, not the individual. In fact, the focus is taken away from weight entirely. Rather than weight loss as a goal, it is process-focused and acknowledges that well-being is dynamic, not fixed.

The weight-inclusive approach goes by several other names, including Health At Every Size (HAES®) or a non-diet approach.

I'll say it again: a HAES® approach does not focus on weight. Instead, weight loss is placed on the back burner and people are encouraged to be kinder to themselves, accept their bodies as they are, and engage in health-promoting behaviours such as physical activity and eating a balanced diet as a form of self-care. HAES® is not suggesting you are healthy at every size, or that everyone can be healthy at any size. That is not what it means at all. Instead, it is promoting health behaviours at whatever size you happen to be right now. Whether you're a size 8 or size 28, you can benefit from healthy behaviours.

The evidence suggests it works. Following the HAES® approach leads to improvements in physiological markers of health such as blood pressure, improvements in health-promoting behaviours, increased self-esteem and reduced disordered eating. The HAES® approach achieves these improvements in health more successfully than weight-focused approaches,[2] with no adverse outcomes. Contrast this with all the known side effects of dieting and focusing on weight loss.

In one particular study, a weight-inclusive programme was evaluated against a weight-loss programme with adult overweight women. All participants had weekly group sessions. The weight-inclusive programme showed better results after one year and again after two years of follow-up.[18] The HAES® group had lower cholesterol levels, lower blood lipid levels and lower blood pressure – all important biomarkers of health. The dieting group did lose weight and showed some improvements after one year, but these were not sustained after two years. The participants had regained the weight they lost and did not maintain the improvements in biomarkers. On top of that, the HAES® group showed reduced body dissatisfaction, perceived hunger, disordered eating symptoms and depression. Their self-esteem had increased, and they were happier and more in tune with their bodies, regardless of whether they had lost weight or not.

Overall, a HAES® approach seems to produce better and longer-lasting health benefits than weight-loss-focused approaches. By not relying on weight as a marker for health, individuals are less likely to be discouraged if their weight doesn't change. This way they're more likely to focus on behaviours that are beneficial to health, rather than potentially growing discouraged and abandoning healthy behaviours in favour of focusing on weight.

The dietary component of HAES® is based on a model of intuitive eating. This is a 10-step process that focuses on internal body awareness, rather than relying on external factors to tell you when, what and how much to eat. Instead of an app, a diet plan or the scales dictating your eating habits, your cues come from your body itself. If you think about it, this makes logical sense. Hundreds of years ago we didn't have such in-depth knowledge about calories and energy, we didn't weigh ourselves and we didn't have apps tracking everything we do. Of course, our food environment was different back then, and that absolutely plays a role, but we also listened to our bodies more. From an evolutionary perspective of basic survival, it makes sense for our bodies to 'know' approximately how much food we need. We experience sensations of hunger and fullness for that reason. Our hunger signals indicate we need energy, and our fullness signals indicate when it's time to stop.

Evidence shows greater well-being for those who can recognise and respond to physiological hunger and fullness cues to determine how much and when to eat, and for those who pay attention to how foods affect their body. These people are more able to adapt to the food environment.

Of course, it's never completely that simple. Years of dieting and ignoring these cues can erode them. Lack of sleep can also disrupt hunger/fullness cues as it interferes with the body's hunger hormone levels, particularly leptin and ghrelin.[42] (We'll be touching much more on sleep and its role in health later on.) But this doesn't mean that you can't relearn to listen and respond to these cues. It's absolutely possible.

Intuitive eaters have been shown to have better mental health, body appreciation, positive emotional functioning, life satisfaction, blood cholesterol levels and blood pressure, and eat a greater variety of foods. Intuitive eating is pretty amazing, and if you want to learn more about how you can get started with it... Well, you'll have to wait until the last chapter. I promise it's worth the wait.

Critics of the non-diet approach have expressed concern that encouraging people to accept their bodies leads them to eat with complete disregard for nutritional considerations, and that due to the abundant food environment this would lead to weight gain. An understandable position, as it can be hard to imagine why someone would want to eat well if there's no one cracking the whip. But this isn't what the evidence shows. No randomised controlled study on HAES® has resulted in weight gain, and rather than people eating worse diets, it actually leads to better dietary quality and eating behaviour.[2] This is in direct contrast to dieting behaviour, which is associated with weight gain over time.

There is an underlying belief that careful monitoring of food intake is essential for keeping appetite under control, and that people would make nutritionally poor choices or eat to excess without monitoring. However, eating restraint is linked to weight gain over time.[7] In contrast, intuitive eating is associated with improved nutrient intake and reduced eating disorder symptoms, not with weight gain.[43]

Framing self-acceptance as 'promoting obesity' misses the point entirely as it is not evidence-based, is stigmatising, and is just plain wrong. Encouraging people to be happier in their own bodies means people are more likely to take care of their bodies and engage in positive health behaviours. Think of how you treat your favourite possessions, or how children look after their favourite toy so carefully. If we can see our body as something to accept and nourish and care for rather than something to fight and insult, then we will do things for it that help it thrive.

I'm a very cynical, sarcastic person, and I'll admit the whole notion of self-acceptance and self-love put me off at the start because it just seemed so corny and woo. But if I can get past that idea and appreciate the evidence and logic behind the argument, then so can you.

Within a HAES® approach, the goal with movement is to promote well-being and self-care rather than prescriptive frequency and duration of exercise. Being active is promoted for its numerous health benefits independent of weight loss. What are those benefits? You'll have to wait until Chapter 8 to find out.

The weight-inclusive approach may seem radical, but seeing as it follows a path that doesn't end up doing more harm than good, and is more sustainable long term, it does make more sense.

Conclusion

Overall, we know that dieting and focusing on weight loss is not sustainable over time for the vast majority of people, and is linked to a range of seriously harmful consequences. This approach is neither ethical nor effective, and we really need to rethink the way we approach the conversation around weight.

The main message I want you to take away from this is that weight and health aren't as synonymous as we might have been led to believe. Weight is not the be-all and end-all. There is so much more to health than just weight. We know that encouraging healthy behaviours improves people's lives regardless of whether they lose weight or not. We know that weight loss diets are highly unsuccessful and demotivating. When we focus on weight we inadvertently encourage disordered eating behaviours and stigmatise people for the way they look. This then has the opposite effect to what is intended – it leads to weight gain, not weight loss, and definitely not health gain.

The bottom line is this: you cannot tell how healthy someone is by their weight. So let's be a little kinder to ourselves and each other, and not make judgements based on appearance.

Quiz: Check your weight bias

Please indicate how much you agree or disagree with each of the following statements:

	STRONGLY DISAGREE	DISAGREE	NEITHER AGREE NOR DISAGREE	AGREE	STRONGLY AGREE
Fat people are less physically attractive than thin people.	1	2	3	4	5
I would never date a fat person.	1	2	3	4	5
On average, fat people are lazier than thin people.	1	2	3	4	5
Fat people only have themselves to blame for their weight.	1	2	3	4	5
It is disgusting when a fat person wears a bathing suit at the beach.	1	2	3	4	5

The higher your total score, the stronger your negative attitudes are towards fat people. Ideally you want this score to be as low as possible, so if you have a high score maybe this is something you can work on.

3

EMOTIONAL EATING

*'When people turn to food and they're not physically
hungry, it means that they're using food for something
else besides satisfying the needs of the body. They're
using it for a different kind of hunger - an emotional
hunger, a psychological hunger, or a spiritual hunger.'*

GENEEN ROTH

We all have an emotional relationship with food – it's part
of being human. Emotional eating is the act of using
food to make yourself feel better. We humans are emotional
beings and don't just eat to satisfy physical hunger; we also eat
to satisfy our emotional needs. Generally, we eat emotionally
in response to negative emotions such as stress or loneliness,
rather than positive ones such as happiness. This is something
we're taught from birth – as babies our first experience of
eating or feeding is connected to being held by a parent, so
we start to equate food with comfort and safety. These early
experiences shape our understanding of how food is connected
to emotion.

How do you know if you're emotional eating? Here are some ways you might be able to identify it:

- Emotional hunger comes on suddenly rather than slowly. It feels like an itch that urgently needs scratching.
- You crave very specific foods, such as pizza or chocolate.
- You don't eat mindfully, despite a lack of distractions.
- You really want to eat even though you feel totally full and satisfied.
- Emotional hunger often leads to regret, guilt or shame.

These aren't foolproof rules, though: sometimes physical hunger can feel sudden if you've been totally distracted by something like work or seeing your favourite band live. Sometimes you have specific cravings because your body knows exactly what nutrients it wants; you may still crave something sweet after dinner because it's a habit you've developed; and there is a whole host of reasons why you might feel guilty for eating something (of course, guilt is never an ideal response to food!). However, these are some useful guidelines to illustrate the idea that emotional eating is different from eating in response to hunger.

Emotional eating gets a bad rep. It's seen as a sign of weakness, a lack of willpower, an inability to 'control our emotions'. But I think it's important not to dismiss emotional eating in this way, and instead to understand the origins and mechanisms behind it. After all, our mental and emotional health is just as important as our physical health.

It probably goes without saying that happiness is important for our health. If we're healthy we're more likely to be happier, but the reverse relationship is also true, and happiness has significant impacts on our health. Being happier means we're more likely to be healthier for longer. There are strong associations in the scientific literature between low happiness and future development of heart disease, stroke, suicide, and early death in general. Happier people live longer, and they have stronger immune systems, better circulatory systems and endocrine (hormone) systems. Happier people are less likely, for example, to catch a cold, and also recover faster if they do catch one.[44]

But what role does food play in our happiness and our mental well-being? Think back to the last time you felt sad, happy, stressed or lonely. I'll bet food was involved in some way. Food can impact our mood, and our mood can influence our food choices. Understanding the impact food can have on our mood can help us to become happier and healthier as a result.

The most obvious example known to most of us is the idea of 'comfort food' – foods that satisfy an emotional as well as a physical need. Comfort foods are a legitimate thing and have been studied by researchers in a variety of settings. The foods we perceive as comfort foods vary from person to person, as they are dependent on our upbringing, our culture, and our experiences growing up. What is consistent, though, is the effect comfort food can have on our emotional state. Food can help alleviate negative emotions such as stress, loneliness, anger and depression.

Stress

Stress is a process by which any challenging experience or event, whether emotional or physiological, results in changes in the body to try to re-establish normality or stability. Emotional stressors are what we most commonly think of as stressful events, such as going through a break-up, the death of a family member, or unemployment. Physiological stressors include starvation, sleep deprivation, severe illness and hyper- or hypothermia.

Stressful experiences can therefore be emotionally or physiologically challenging. Stress changes our eating patterns and affects appetite through the hormones that are produced as a result of the stress response. The most important of these hormones are: cortisol, adrenaline and noradrenaline.

A note on hormones

Before we get into the nitty-gritty of the stress response, a quick word on hormones.

Hormones are the chemical messengers sent out by your endocrine system. They travel around the body via your bloodstream to send signals to various target organs and tissues in order to get your body to do something, such as changing blood pressure or initiating a behaviour. Every multicellular organism has hormones. They are involved in every system in the body, including the ones we're focusing on here: stress and appetite.

- Ghrelin – the hunger hormone. It is made in the stomach.
- Leptin – reduces hunger. It is made by cells in fat tissue.
- Neuropeptide Y – increases hunger and reduces anxiety. It is made in the stomach.

- Insulin – controls blood glucose (blood sugar) levels. It is made by the pancreas.
- Cortisol – also known as the stress hormone. It is made in the adrenal cortex, part of the adrenal gland.
- Adrenaline (also known as epinephrine) – part of the 'fight or flight' response. It is made in the adrenal medulla, part of the adrenal gland.
- Noradrenaline (also known as norepinephrine) – part of the 'fight or flight' response. It is made in the adrenal medulla, part of the adrenal gland.

In humans, the stress response is manifested through two interacting stress pathways: the hypothalamic-pituitary-adrenal (HPA) axis and the sympathetic-adrenal medullary (SAM) system. The HPA axis is a neuroendocrine system and communication pathway between the hypothalamus in the brain, the pituitary gland in the brain, and the adrenal glands above the kidneys. In the HPA axis, stress stimulates the release of a hormone from the hypothalamus, which stimulates the synthesis of another hormone from the pituitary, which triggers production of glucocorticoids (mainly cortisol) from the adrenal cortex. So, in plain English, stress stimulates a signalling cascade from your brain to the adrenal glands that results in cortisol release. Which is why cortisol is commonly referred to as the stress hormone.

The SAM system is activated in response to acute stress, which triggers the release of the hormones adrenaline and noradrenaline. These hormones promote energy responses in the body, such as increased cardiac output, blood pressure and triglyceride levels, and redirection of blood to fuel the muscles, heart and brain. Overall, this promotes the fight-or-flight

response. Systems that might compete for energy, such as repro-
duction and digestion, are inhibited – meaning that the acute
stress response includes suppressing appetite and food intake.
This is a feeling we can probably all relate to; for example, you
may find that during a stressful exam you don't feel hungry at
all, then as soon as you put down your pen and leave the room,
your stomach starts rumbling. I don't imagine many people
would feel hungry if you're on a plane that's experiencing
heavy turbulence, or when you're walking home alone late at
night. During acutely stressful times – which in the past would
be more likely to feature being chased or attacked by a wild
animal – it's more helpful for your appetite to be suppressed, as
it would otherwise provide a distraction when you need to focus
and either face the fear (fight) or get away from it as quickly as
possible (flight).

Acute stress can be beneficial and activate responses in the
body that help you get through that stressful situation, whereas
prolonged chronic stress leads to wear and tear of the body's
regulatory systems. Repeated and uncontrollable stress can
dysregulate the HPA axis over time, which then affects energy
balance and eating behaviours. Chronic stress can also weaken
any beneficial responses to stress, dampen the immune system
and lead to increased risk of disease.

These two systems, the HPA axis and the SAM system, release
hormones that affect our appetite hormones. Both systems
result in release of glucocorticoids, of which cortisol is the most
famous one. High cortisol in the bloodstream increases leptin,
ghrelin and neuropeptide Y. Leptin inhibits appetite, ghrelin
increases appetite, and neuropeptide Y increases appetite as
well as specifically making us crave carbs. Also, noradrenaline

tends to suppress appetite during stress, whereas cortisol tends to stimulate appetite during recovery from stress. Some of these effects seem to be directly contradictory, so what effect does this swirling hormone soup actually have on you, the person?

Stress itself alters metabolism independent of a person's lifestyle habits.[45] Around 40 per cent of people increase their caloric intake when stressed, 40 per cent decrease, and around 20 per cent don't change behaviours during stressful times.[46] Over 70 per cent of us are also more likely to snack when we're stressed and less likely to eat proper meals. These individual differences partly depend on what's causing stress, how long that stress lasts and how hungry someone is to begin with. Mild stressors seem to lead to increased food intake, whereas more severe stressors lead to decreased intake. For some people, stress doesn't seem to have any significant effect on their eating at all! Although there are differences across the population, what appears to be the case is that people don't fluctuate between eating more in response to stress one week, then eating less the week after. We're consistent in our responses, so if you're the kind of person who eats more when stressed, then that's unlikely to change over time.

If you're someone who eats more in response to stress, then you likely have high stress reactivity – meaning you show a stronger cortisol increase in response to stress, which drives your appetite hormones up and encourages you to eat.[47] People who experience high stress reactivity may choose energy-dense foods to blunt the stress response or reduce anxiety. Given that we live in a food environment where we have an abundance of energy-dense food that is readily available and easily accessible, this is an understandable response to stress.

Although stress leads to increased leptin levels, which you would expect to decrease appetite, instead it seems that the large amounts of glucocorticoids decrease our sensitivity to leptin, meaning that we need much larger amounts of leptin to have the same response to it. So, although we have plenty of appetite-suppressing leptin around, the body doesn't respond to it, and so our appetite doesn't go down. This occurs in individuals across the BMI spectrum.[47]

As well as quantity of food, stress can also affect our specific food preferences and choices. Stress is associated with a shift towards choosing more palatable, delicious foods, regardless of change in total energy intake. These foods tend to be both high in fat and high in sugar,[48] particularly desserts and snacks, as these are especially delicious to us. When experiencing stress, most people tend to choose foods that taste sweet.[49]

Overall, we can conclude that stress has a pretty detrimental effect on our eating patterns. Not only are we far more likely to overeat, snack more, and go for high-sugar, high-fat foods, stress is also linked to binge-eating in some people. It should be noted that these effects are consistent across genders.

High levels of stress can alter the body's ability to regulate appetite and energy, which can lead to overeating as the body is unable to send you the proper signals to say, 'Stop eating, I'm full'. Over time, chronic stress is therefore linked to weight gain. High stress and high cortisol levels also affect insulin. This hormone is normally released by the pancreas into the blood-stream in response to you eating glucose (and some protein), which then encourages glucose to be taken up by cells to be used for energy. Think of it this way: every cell has a door that only glucose can go through, and insulin is the key that unlocks that door. Without insulin, glucose just stays in the bloodstream and your cells can't use it for energy. Cortisol messes with insulin by preventing secretion from the pancreas and preventing cells from creating enough doors to allow glucose through. So we end up with a lack of keys and a lack of doors. This can lead to insulin resistance – the precursor to type 2 diabetes.[47]

Before, I mentioned that our stress responses are pretty consistent; however, one factor does seem to change this: dieting. Dieting or restrained eating is associated with increased cortisol, and may increase your vulnerability towards stress-induced increased appetite. So, if you're usually the kind of person who's not that affected by stress but you decide to go on a diet, you may then suddenly start overeating in response to stress. In fact, it's been suggested that this is why there is such a divide in terms of stress-induced appetite responses: those who are dieting generally eat more when stressed, those who aren't on diets generally don't. It has been estimated that around 70 per cent of those who eat more when stressed are restrained eaters or are on a diet.[48]

Restraint may be associated with greater food intake following stress, but in these people, emotional eating is only linked to eating more in response to an ego threat – a threat to a person's self-image or self-esteem. This means restraint may encourage eating in response to stimuli such as stress, whereas emotional eating tries to cancel out negative self-focused emotions.

People who are on diets tend to have rigid rules around their eating habits – what they are and aren't allowed to eat, for example – and so are less tuned in to the physiological cues of hunger and satiety, which can also lead to overeating.

It has been suggested that people on a diet are so focused on maintaining restraint and control around food that they don't have the emotional energy to deal with stressors, and so end up overeating; or that their self-imposed restriction breaks down in favour of dealing with a more urgent concern (the stress).

The particular foods that are commonly chosen when stressed, such as sweets or crisps, are also often foods that people avoid when they're on a diet as they are 'forbidden' foods. It's interesting that people on a diet are far more likely to increase their intake of these foods when stressed, as these are foods that are not typically 'allowed'. They reportedly eat these foods to make themselves feel better.[48] This can go part way towards explaining why dieting is a risk factor for weight gain, and why diets tend to fail. People typically describe experiencing short-term loss in appetite, and possibly some weight loss, in response to stress, followed by a compensatory increase in appetite once the stressful situation has passed, which leads to weight regain, sometimes to a higher weight than before. In addition, regular chronic stress (even just five days a week) and its disruption to the body's appetite signals can exacerbate this further.

Low stress levels and the ability to cope well in stressful situations goes a long way towards maintaining a stable weight, rather than fluctuation and weight-cycling, which, as discussed in the previous chapter, is not a good place to be in. In addition, it's worth noting that experiencing weight stigma would be considered a stressor, and if experienced regularly can lead to chronic stress, again supporting the argument that shaming people into losing weight is not the answer.

High levels of stress increase consumption of highly palatable foods, so it makes sense that high levels of stress can affect the brain reward systems. Activation of the HPA axis is linked to activation of the dopamine reward system in the brain, as both food and food cues increase dopamine release. But it's important to note that dopamine release is not equivalent to addictive properties. The hormones involved in appetite and energy balance, such as leptin and ghrelin, can also play a role in food cravings. This is important as it provides a link between high levels of cortisol (stress), increased appetite, and increased desire to eat highly palatable foods that activate the reward centres in the brain (and therefore make you feel better). These foods produce a response in the brain that helps calm down the HPA axis, thereby reducing the stress response.[50] So consuming these kinds of foods actually helps to reduce stress on a biochemical level. Amazing!

Chronic stress is often accompanied by other emotions such as anxiety, depression, anger, apathy and loneliness. Hyperpalatable foods may serve as 'comfort foods' as a form of self-medication to alleviate these feelings of distress. This adds an additional psychological component to what is otherwise a very physiological argument for emotional eating. Let's look at this idea of comfort foods in a bit more depth in connection with another strong emotion: loneliness.

Loneliness

Moving away from home, fighting with a close friend, breaking up with a partner, and many other similar circumstances can leave people feeling alone and isolated. When these situations occur, the comfort of a familiar food can be especially enticing.

Comfort food helps alleviate loneliness, as these foods are associated with specific people and our relationships with them. As humans, we are desperate to belong and to form relationships with people, to the point where it's been argued to be a fundamental human need. We want to avoid feeling lonely. Feeling lonely and being socially isolated is both physically and psychologically damaging, as it can lead to lowered self-esteem, depression, and even physical sensations of pain.[51]

Recent research suggests that people sometimes seek out 'social surrogates' when they want to avoid feeling lonely. These can be in the form of escaping into the world of a fantasy novel, writing in a diary or seeking out food. Comfort food is one way in which people can find a sense of belonging in the midst of their loneliness. While comfort foods are associated with happy times, they are almost exclusively eaten alone, not with others. It has been suggested that foods become comfort food because of the associations with specific people or occasions, and those associations get reinforced to the point where that food reminds you of someone or something every time you eat it. In one study, comfort foods were usually identified as a family tradition, a cultural tradition, something eaten for a holiday, or a reminder of home.[51] They were not usually typical everyday foods. Christmas dinner is an excellent example of this. If you close your eyes and imagine last year's Christmas dinner, does it make you feel warm and happy inside? I bet it does.

Four types of comfort food have been identified: nostalgic foods, indulgence foods, convenience foods and physical comfort foods.[52] Many foods can also fall into more than one category.

Nostalgic foods

These are foods that remind you of moments in your own history, especially from childhood. A particular food may remind you of something you used to bake together with your mother, or a weekend childhood family tradition, or a meal you'd share with your dad when you spent time together one-to-one. When you feel lonely or disconnected from people you love, eating foods that reminds you of them can help bring them closer, so they don't feel so far away, especially in unfamiliar surroundings. Nostalgic foods, especially ones linked to childhood, evoke feelings of being cared for by someone, particularly our mothers. This is obviously conditional on having a happy childhood with a caring mother. These foods are also linked to sharing food with loved ones, particularly sharing of family meals around the dinner table on special occasions, and the preparation of food. Nostalgic foods are less likely to be takeaways or ready meals, instead leaning more towards meals cooked from scratch in a family kitchen. Preparing food with someone and spending time in the kitchen together is quite an intimate thing – I'm sure you'd be happy to invite new acquaintances into your dining or living room but be more hesitant about having them in your kitchen, especially while you're cooking. It's the 'behind the scenes' part that only the lucky few generally get to see.

There's a reason that comfort foods tend to be foods we're already familiar with. New foods just don't feel the same, and from an evolutionary perspective, new foods were potential sources of danger, whereas familiar foods were safe – you knew they wouldn't kill you! So whereas new foods can evoke feelings of anxiety, familiar foods can help relieve feelings of distress.

Indulgence foods

These tend to be foods that are often perceived as 'unhealthy' or high in calories. They can be comforting to someone, as they are often foods high in fat and sugar, which makes them particularly palatable and incredibly delicious, lighting up pleasure centres in the brain. Research shows that concerns about nutrition, while noted, get ignored in favour of making a food choice that would satisfy cravings and improve mood.[52] A sentiment I think we can all relate to! Indulgence foods are also often used to provide comfort when trying to get through difficult challenges, such as exams, stressful times at work, or even just feeling tired and hungover. Takeaway pizza is a wonderful example of this, as is reaching for baked goods as a reward for having finished an evening of overtime, or using sweets to help teach your child maths. In this way, indulgence foods can also be a security blanket during times of low self-esteem. In addition, an interesting explanation for indulgence foods as comfort foods is that we crave these foods because we restrict them. Restriction almost inevitably leads to overeating and feeling strong negative emotions such as sadness or loneliness makes that restriction and 'willpower' to avoid them so much harder. So we don't avoid them, and reach for them to help us feel better.

Convenience foods

These are pretty self-explanatory. When you're feeling down, lonely or stressed, you want something that'll make you feel better immediately. No preparation, no cooking and no effort.

If you're feeling sad, sometimes even something as simple as cooking can feel too much. You want effortless gratification, and convenience foods provide just that.

Physical comfort foods

These provide comfort by passing on their physical attributes to you, the person eating them. An 'icy stare' is not literally icy, but it can send a cold shiver down your spine. Similarly, a warm, comforting meal can produce a feeling almost like an internal hug. It warms up the body and fills you up, removing feelings of emptiness. In this way, comfort foods provide both physical and psychological comfort.

Interestingly, there seem to be some differences in comfort food preferences across ages and genders. Men, and those who identify as male, are more likely to reach for warm, hearty meals, whereas women, and those who identify as female, are more likely to reach for sweet foods and snacks.[53] Younger people also generally prefer more snacks, whereas older people prefer whole meals. In both women and younger people in general, eating these foods is associated with more feelings of guilt for 'giving in' to these cravings.

Anger

Anger is not seen as a productive or acceptable emotion; it's a 'bad' feeling that has to be channelled into something more 'positive'. This is particularly so for women, who are often not allowed to express anger in society and told to 'calm down' instead, as it's seen as too aggressive and masculine. So because anger cannot be expressed outwardly at the source, it's directed either inwardly or towards food – hence why women tend to feel a stronger desire to eat in response to anger compared with men.[54] Keeping such an emotion inside can be uncomfortable, and so comfort foods are sought out to negate the discomfort. Food is also a distraction, as anger is an emotion that is usually followed by an action of some sort, and the action of eating allows us to move away from these feelings of anger.

Particularly for those who have issues with conflict, feeling angry can be a scary experience, and so food is used to bury those feelings, thereby avoiding any conflict. Eating in response to anger can also lead someone to feel angry and frustrated with themselves for feeling out of control, which directs the anger away from someone or something else and towards themselves instead. This is more common if they are someone who has depression, low self-esteem, or generally has a habit of thinking very negatively about themselves – blaming yourself is a much more comfortable and familiar place to be.

Anger drives us to eat more impulsively, meaning fast and irregular eating directed at any food type available.[55] Being 'hangry' (hungry-angry) is an interesting phenomenon as well, although it's more likely to be irritability than pure anger. Being hungry can influence mood, for example through the release of cortisol and adrenaline, which make you feel more tense. On top of that, low blood sugar is also a pretty unpleasant feeling. Interestingly though, we're more likely to experience hanger if we're unaware that we're physiologically hungry, which sounds the wrong way round. Feeling hangry occurs when your hunger-induced negativity gets blamed on external factors, like the person who stole your parking space or suddenly stopped directly in front of you while walking. You assume they're the ones who are making you angry, not the fact that you're super hungry. But this isn't a deliberate process; it's unconscious.[56]

Being overly hungry/hangry can not only just lead to you snapping at someone unnecessarily but can also easily lead to overeating, as we tend to eat more quickly with less thought, and are less likely to pause partway through eating. Paying more attention to hunger is the key here.

Boredom

A brief word on boredom. Boredom can be described as 'emotional purgatory'. It's neither a good mood nor a bad mood, it's just there. It's meh. It's the emoji of the person shrugging with indifference. As a result, it hasn't been studied to the same extent that stress and loneliness have in relation to eating.

We are all likely to eat more when we're bored. Very strong, powerful emotions, such as heightened anxiety, rage or acute stress, tend to reduce our food intake, whereas more mellow emotions like boredom increase our chances of overeating. In fact, food is often the first thing we think of in relation to boredom, unlike other emotions.[57] How many times have you been bored at home and walked over to your fridge, opened it, stared inside, maybe picked at something and then left again, only to repeat this same process a few minutes later?

Unlike stress eating or eating due to loneliness, boredom eating feels pretty pointless. We usually boredom-eat when we don't actually physically need food, and there's something more useful we could be doing. So in some ways it's a form of procrastination. After a few bites the food usually isn't even that satisfying, as we weren't actually hungry to begin with.

Why do we eat when we're bored? It's worth pointing out that sometimes boredom allows us to realise that we are genuinely physically hungry. Sometimes we can be so focused on work or a video game or a book that we tune out our hunger signals, and then boredom allows them to become the focus again. But for those situations when you're not actually physically hungry, it may simply be that we're willing to do anything to avoid boredom (even give ourselves electric shocks![58]) and food is just a nice, convenient way to do that.

It may also link back to dopamine and the reward system in our brain. We are evolutionarily programmed to enjoy food. Food is supposed to elicit a pleasure response in our brains. While this is a distinct advantage – it makes food more enjoyable and so we eat it and don't starve to death – it can also have its downsides.

It's possible that when we're feeling bored and unmotivated, so are our dopamine neurons. When we eat out of boredom, what we're really doing is trying to get them awake and excited again. In the absence of any other dopamine trigger, food looks like a pretty effective and easy way of doing that.

This also goes some way towards explaining why we tend to reach for snacks and sweet treats when we're bored, rather than full meals. Some people, of course, will go hardcore in the kitchen in response to boredom, spending hours baking bread, making cakes or cooking an elaborate feast. But generally we want something quick to distract us from boredom, or to procrastinate and give us a little pleasure hit before getting back to what we need to be doing.

I would go so far as to suggest this isn't an inherently bad thing. Sometimes a little break and burst of pleasure is ideal for getting us into a better mindset to just get shit done. But if it's a regular repetitive habit, it can lead to overeating, feelings of guilt and stress.

Happiness

We have enough evidence to say that negative emotions cause increased food intake in a great many people.[59] But food doesn't just help us get out of a negative place, it can also help us feel happier in general. In the short term, comfort foods are very much what we lean towards, as they provide an immediate alleviation of negative mood. This is exactly what we need at that moment in time, and there's absolutely nothing wrong with that. In the long term, however, the kind of patterns of eating that promote lasting happiness are ones based on plenty of fruits and vegetables.[49] Not only that, but foods rich in carbohydrates are known to increase serotonin levels in the brain, and as serotonin is also known as the 'happy hormone', yes, that means carbohydrates make you happier.[60] Serotonin is made from the amino acid tryptophan*, but ironically, consumption of high-protein foods actually decreases the level of tryptophan and serotonin in the brain, whereas carbohydrates increase levels. When you eat

---

* Amino acids are the building blocks of protein, and so you'd assume that high protein foods would give you the highest amount of tryptophan.

high-protein foods, tryptophan competes with other amino acids to get past the blood-brain barrier into the brain, and all that competition means less tryptophan makes it through, and you don't get such an increase in serotonin. However, when you eat carbohydrates, insulin is released, which triggers most amino acids to be absorbed into the bloodstream, and tryptophan has a free ride up into the brain, where it increases serotonin levels. But not all carbohydrates affect serotonin equally: it's the complex carbohydrates found in vegetables and whole grains that seem to improve mood, more so than simple sugars. I find this ironic, considering a number of celebrity chefs and gym bros have made good money by telling people that the diet that makes you happy is a low-carb diet high in protein and fat. It is true, though, that dopamine levels are increased by eating protein-rich foods, and while dopamine doesn't have the same effects as serotonin, it does contribute to overall mood and well-being. Obviously, we don't eat carbohydrates or protein in isolation, we eat foods that contain these nutrients, so overall the key (food-wise) to long-term happiness lies in a healthy, balanced diet that includes sources of protein and carbohydrates.

This whole concept links beautifully back to the chapter on weight and health: if we are kind to our body, we are more likely to treat it well by feeding it a well-balanced diet, which will in turn make us happier.

Knowing that foods make us happier, the next step would be assessing if food can help with depression. There is a clear link between diet and risk of depression. Broadly speaking, people who eat a wide variety of fruits, vegetables, nuts and oily fish (all nutrient-dense foods) have a reduced risk of depression.[61] The difficulty here is that the relationship seems to go both ways: if you're depressed, you're less likely to cook and feed yourself well by following a well-balanced, nutrient-dense diet, and if you don't eat well that can impact your mood so you feel worse. But you may have spotted that this nutrient-dense diet is very much the Mediterranean way of eating. Following a Mediterranean-style diet can help alleviate the symptoms of depression, more so than social interactions.[62] So we can now say that eating well causes an improvement in symptoms of depression.

Considering depression is such a serious issue, this could have serious implications for treatment. Dietary improvement may provide an efficacious and accessible treatment strategy for the management of depression. But I have to stress that studies examined the effects of diet on depression alongside standard treatment. Food was not, and should not, be used as a stand-alone treatment for depression. It should only be considered in addition to talking therapy or medication (or both) that it should be considered. It would also be misleading and unethical to suggest that eating a nutrient-poor diet causes depression, because that absolutely isn't the case. Depression is complex and multifactorial, often linked to trauma, stressful life events, abuse or brain chemistry. While consuming nutrient-dense foods may help with symptoms, this will not be addressing the underlying cause.

We have a tendency to focus on the aspects of foods that affect our physical health, and not the emotional aspects. But food is so much more than just fuel; food nourishes your mind as well as your body. We all have an emotional connection with food, and that's backed up by the research out there right now. There are some physiological reasons why these foods make us feel good: high-carbohydrate foods can increase serotonin levels in the brain, and highly palatable foods activate the reward centres in our brains. But these reasons aren't enough to explain the existence of comfort foods. They don't explain the diversity in foods identified as comfort foods, explain why we choose some and not others, and why we choose certain foods in particular situations.

Diet quality and nutrition are clearly important factors in mental health. There's no denying that reconciling negative feelings and emotions by eating comfort foods can be riskier than other methods of dealing with these emotions, as it can lead to overeating or disordered eating patterns. But it's far from the worst coping mechanism, as I'd argue using drugs or alcohol poses more serious health risks. While there is nothing inherently wrong with using food to help soothe emotions – it's totally normal and part of being human – it can become a problem if food is the only coping strategy you have.

I want to be absolutely clear that it is totally normal to eat for emotional reasons. I also want to point out that there will be times when we think we're emotional eating, but actually we may just be hungry. If you eat an apple for breakfast and a small salad for lunch, then you get home and demolish the entire contents of the fridge, that's not emotional eating. You were just really hungry and needed to eat! Making sure you're eating enough throughout the day is one easy way to prevent some cases of emotional eating – being super hungry is a stressful state for your body – as is taking time to de-stress, and having other coping mechanisms available to you when you experience negative emotions.

In short, it's an oversimplification to dismiss emotional eating as 'unhealthy'. It's more nuanced than that.

Quiz: How is your emotional eating?

All of us respond to different emotions in different ways, and sometimes those feelings make us want to eat. Please indicate the extent to which each of the following feelings leads you to feel an urge to eat by checking the appropriate box.

	NO DESIRE TO EAT	A SMALL DESIRE TO EAT	A MODERATE DESIRE TO EAT	A STRONG DESIRE TO EAT	AN OVER-WHELMING DESIRE TO EAT
Inadequate					
Excited					
Sad					
Irritated					
Jealous					
Worried					
Frustrated					
Lonely					
Stressed					
Angry					
Nervous					
Guilty					
Bored					
Helpless					
Upset					
Happy					

The more your answers are over to the right side of the table, the more you are driven to eat in response to emotions. This is not a diagnostic tool but is here to help you recognise and gain awareness of your current response to emotional situations. The final chapter offers some guidance on strategies to ensure you don't rely so heavily on food as a tool.

4

CLEANING UP THE LANGUAGE OF FOOD

'You are what you eat, so don't be fast, cheap, easy or fake.'

THE INTERNET

'You are what you eat, so own it and enjoy it.'

ME

Imagine eating a burger, fries and a milkshake. What words and emotions spring to mind when you think about this scenario? Some might say 'delicious', 'treats', 'indulgence'. Many would probably say 'unhealthy', 'guilt', 'shame', 'regret', 'fattening' or 'gross'.

The language we use to describe food is important, but it's something that doesn't get talked about enough. The way we eat is part of our identity, because the food we eat *becomes* us: our bones, our muscles, our adipose tissue, our neurons - everything. Everything we eat is converted into our bodies.

So, by that extension, the way we describe food and the way we feel about food is mimicked in the way we feel about ourselves. If we use negative language to describe food, we attribute those words to ourselves as well, and considering most of the population has a negative body image, we don't need to add to this.

Having negative associations with foods can lead to feelings of anxiety or guilt at having eaten them, as well as thoughts of how to compensate for this behaviour: skipping the next meal, eating a lot less the next day, doing an extra workout or even purging. These are not healthy food behaviours.

The language we use to describe food affects not only us but also those within earshot of our conversations. Loudly proclaiming, 'Oh God, I'm being so bad today by eating this cake' may decrease not only your enjoyment of the cake, but also that of the person sitting at the next table, who, up until that point, was feeling totally fine about eating cake. If someone near you is more vulnerable to these kinds of comments, you could be negatively affecting their mental health.

Some of the words we so easily use to describe food could very well be having a detrimental effect on our health. In our quest to be healthy, we often use very unhealthy language. This is especially the case in the diet industry. There is a fine line between promoting a healthy diet (a good thing) and causing anxiety over foods (definitely not good).

We can't escape metaphors in our lives. For example, money is used as a metaphorical source for time: we spend time, save time, and waste it. This in turn affects how we perceive time and how we behave towards it – we act as if time is something tangible, valuable, measurable and divisible. Motivational videos will take this one step further and tell you that if you received £86,400 every day, how would you spend it, knowing it would disappear at the end of the day? You wouldn't waste it, so why are you wasting the 86,400 seconds you have every day of your life? It implies that each second is equally valuable.

We use the language of eating as a metaphor for how we interact with the world around us. For example:

- 'You look so pretty I could just eat you up.'
- 'He has bitten off more than he can chew.'
- 'I am always hungry for new experience.'
- 'A feast for the eyes.'
- 'I have acquired a taste for skiing.'

Desire is hunger, so satisfying desire is eating.[63]

We use food metaphors in everyday life to explain phenomena such as ambition and desire, but we also use religious and moral metaphors and concepts to describe food. As we saw in the first chapter, religious discourse is rife in both the diet and wellness industry, employing words such as 'sinful', 'guilt-free', and 'clean' to provoke feelings of righteousness and/or disgust in eating habits. The best example I can think of is Slimming World and 'syns'. Ugh. What a horrible word, to imply that eating food is a sin.

I want to focus on a few of the terms that I believe should be banished from our vocabulary when it comes to talking about food. I believe these words and phrases have no place in our food conversations, and that despite their potentially harmless appearances, these words are insidious and negatively affect our health.

Clean eating

Clean eating epitomises the idea of 'You are what you eat'. If you eat 'clean' you are a clean person. By extension, if you don't eat 'clean' you must therefore eat dirty and be a dirty person.

The contents of the diet vary from person to person when eating 'clean', and are arguably irrelevant. The term has been adopted so widely, by people promoting so many different eating choices, that it has no agreed-upon definition. I don't care whether eating clean means vegan to one person, avoiding processed foods to another, and eating paleo to a third. What eating clean includes doesn't matter, because it's the very use of language and the morality it imparts on the person that matters here. By simply using the word 'clean', it implies you are therefore better than someone else.

The notions of 'clean' and 'dirty' are strongly tied to notions of right and wrong. Across human societies, bodily purity seems deeply intertwined with morality. You physically wash away your sins to become clean again. I think we can all agree that describing the complexity of sexuality as 'dirty' is neither accurate nor helpful. We recoil at the thought of someone comparing a woman who has had many sexual partners to a dirty stick of gum. We are appalled by this, yet somehow we're supposed to be ok with describing food – another one of life's great pleasures – in similarly loaded terms? I think not.

The 'clean eating' movement used these tactics to fuel the elitism that is rampant in the whole Wellness industry. Wellness puts a price tag on health by making health something only a few people can afford, by making expensive powders seem more desirable, by selling you lies about how if you only eat this way you'll be healthier and superior to others.

While the rules of clean eating can vary from person to person, the underlying commonality is the omission of certain food groups – whether it's gluten, dairy, grains or meat. These are the 'dirty' foods, although they're usually called 'forbidden' foods, whereas foods to include are happily called 'clean'.

'Clean eating' is often associated with thin white women posing on the covers of bestselling books with a plate of vegetables. But the morality of clean eating isn't limited to one gender, although it is marketed differently to men. Rather than the focus being on purity in a feminine sense, instead it is centred on producing a masculine muscular body that is strong and capable. It involves a lifestyle that rejects 'dirty' foods that would pollute or slow down the body and its progress, both in terms of aesthetics (or muscularity) and life ambition/ success.[64]

The idea of 'unclean' foods is physically repulsive to us. If someone served you food on a dirty plate or served you a glass of wine with a lipstick print on it, you'd likely refuse, as the food had been contaminated by the used crockery and was therefore 'impure' and 'unclean'. We feel disgust (a powerful emotion) and that disgust is passed from the plate to the food to the person who eats it. We see this with 'clean eating' as well: people are grossed out by those who eat meat, who eat ready meals, or who eat whatever foods they have deemed to be 'unclean'. The difference, though, is that while the ice cream you dropped in the mud is definitely dirty, the ice cream you've spooned from a mass-produced tub definitely isn't.

By following a 'clean' diet you are therefore proclaiming to the world that you value yourself more highly than someone else, that you take care of yourself better, and that makes you a better person. It's not enough to keep your house clean and maintain personal hygiene; you now also have to be squeaky clean on the inside.

The 'clean eating' movement was very much shot down back in around 2016, and all the wellness bloggers who once used the term have distanced themselves from it, claiming they intended it to mean 'healthy' and they don't like what it's become. In doing so, they not only completely failed to acknowledge that they were the ones who turned the phrase into what it represents, but they also failed to understand the very issue with the word 'clean' – it implies that one person's way of eating makes them morally superior and a better person than another.

Sadly, the phrase, despite being abandoned by those who helped it rise to fame, is still widely used. That needs to stop.

Real food

What is real food? I've yet to come across someone who can define this and who then goes on to actually follow that definition. Most follow the argument of eating only 'whole foods' and nothing processed or anything you can't pronounce. But these same people are usually more than happy to consume protein powders, which are definitely very processed.

Real food doesn't exist. What's the opposite of real food? Fake food – not edible; imaginary food – also not edible. Therefore, surely anything edible is 'real' food? I can hold it in my hands so it must be real. But of course, it's not that simple: 'fake' food is argued to be anything that isn't 'natural' – a word that's even more difficult to define.

'Real' and 'natural' are often used interchangeably when it comes to food, and what is 'real' varies according to the dietary dogma of choice. On many low-carbohydrate diets, 'real food' is generally real fat, and low-fat products are deemed fake and flavourless. Full-fat ice cream is deemed the 'real deal', whereas low-fat ice cream is an 'imitation'. There is a sense that something about the ice cream has been destroyed by removing fat, despite the fact that this is not how low-fat ice cream is made. It implies that food manufacturers start with ordinary ice cream and literally remove the fat from it to distort it into something else. Instead, what actually happens is that they start with different ingredients, such as low-fat dairy products instead of full-fat, and then add additional emulsifiers or other ingredients to improve the texture and 'mouthfeel' to resemble the full-fat version as much as possible. But that truth is pushed aside in favour of the narrative of 'naturalness' and 'wholeness' or inherent integrity that is so important to low-carbohydrate diet discourse.

This idea of 'real food' being 'whole food' also appears in the wellness world, where whole foods are prized above all others, suggesting that other foods are not complete in some way and are (at most) only partially food.

If we then extend this to 'You are what you eat', no one wants to be called fake, whether it's being a 'fake' friend, having a 'fake' designer bag, or being told 'fake news'. It suggests dishonesty, disloyalty, or a malicious intent. 'Real women have curves'... But how can you be a fake woman? Apply this to food and it implies the food has some insidious quality that wants to cause you harm, whereas 'real food' is associated with honesty and pure intentions.

If you want someone to avoid eating something, call it the opposite of 'real food', such as a food-like substance, stuff, product – anything but actual food. We see this in almost every dietary regime under the sun: in low-carbohydrate books, refined carbohydrates are referred to as 'packaged refined carbohydrate stuff'; in the wellness world anything off limits is referred to as 'nasties' or 'empty calories' (see below for more on that one); and in the vegan communities eggs are referred to as 'chicken periods' while meat is 'flesh' to deliberately invoke disgust.

Detox/cleanse

First things first: you have a liver and kidneys, which work hard 24/7 to perform the normal detoxification processes necessary to keep you healthy and alive. No food, no supplement, no special tea can detox your body. You can support your liver by eating a generally well-balanced diet and not binge-drinking, but apart from that the food you eat simply will not detox you.

'Detox' has entered our conversation all too casually, mainly in relation to alcohol. It's also used to mean 'trying to be healthier' or 'trying to lose weight'. 'New year detox'. The popularity of detoxes has come about partly because of a false narrative that modern life is toxic and we have to take additional steps to de-toxify ourselves from all the toxins floating around. We have to purify ourselves, or 'cleanse' our bodies for them to be in their optimum state. This links nicely back to 'eat clean' and is partly why the clean-eating movement is rife with 'detoxing' meals, juices and even juice cleanses. Superfood powders are supposed to help 'detox' you, a 'detox' bowl will supposedly leave you feeling light and fresh rather than sluggish, and juice cleanses allegedly 'reset' your digestion, as if your organs, when malfunctioning, just need to be switched off and back on again like a computer.

It's been suggested that this need to punish ourselves to be healthy, to detox and cleanse ourselves, comes from the fact that many religions practise fasting and purification. And just like holy water purifies you and washes away your sins, so a juice cleanse washes away those pesky toxins that are making you feel run-down, leaving you a purer, better person than you were before (not).

It's fascinating how we use physical cleansing as a coping mechanism and 'cure' for moral impurities. A threat to our moral purity induces the need to cleanse ourselves. In one interesting study, people were asked to recall either an ethical or unethical action from their past. Those who spoke about something unethical they had done were more likely to choose an antiseptic wipe afterwards to wipe their hands with (thereby 'cleansing' themselves) over choosing a pencil (the control item in the study – asking participants to choose between a wipe or nothing wouldn't be a good study design).[65] We can apply that to other behaviours, such as going out drinking at the weekend and maybe saying some things you regret, and feeling the need to go on a juice cleanse on the Monday to wash those negative feelings away.

While this is a possible explanation, many would disagree and think it's simply the dieting industry co-opting religious language to invoke familiarity with a concept, thereby making it more appealing. Because so many of us in our childhood (or adulthood) went to religious services where talk of cleansing was part of the package deal, we see it as familiar and are more drawn to it, and so more likely to buy the products.

So, thinking of a cleanse to atone for last month's dietary sins? Maybe think again.

Cheat meal

Picture the scenario. You've just started on a 'healthy eating' programme, you follow it solidly for 12 weeks, being 'good', being 'disciplined'. Then the 12 weeks are up and you decide you've been so 'good' you deserve a night off. So you have a 'cheat meal' that's definitely not on-plan, and definitely contains forbidden foods. One of two things likely happens: either the 'cheat meal' turns into a 'cheat day' and a 'cheat weekend' and so on, or you overeat, feel guilty and decide to go back to the plan, effectively starting a binge-restrict cycle.

Unsurprisingly, there hasn't been much actual research on 'cheat meals', although one analysis of social media images tagged with #cheatmeal found that a significant number of images showing cheat meals were large enough to be classified as an objective binge.[66] Not even a subjective binge (i.e. a larger-than-usual quantity of food), but an amount of food that would be classified as a binge by the American Psychological Association. That, to me, is very worrying, as it is normalising disordered eating behaviours. The accompanying captions further normalise this, and explicitly refer to compensating for the meal later in the form of exercise, or the meal being a reward for being 'disciplined' for a considerable time before (more on that below). In addition, the foods chosen for a 'cheat meal' tend to be very energy-dense foods like pizza or ice cream, just as is common in an objective binge.

To 'cheat' is to break a rule or 'act dishonestly or unfairly in order to gain an advantage'. What rule are you breaking when you have a cheat meal? It's either one you made up or one given to you by a plan of some sort. In which case it's a diet, and by now I think we've established that diets are not the answer. But even if you don't perceive yourself to be on a diet, this is still the dieting mindset. It's a ridiculously hard mindset to break out of, especially if you've been in the dieting space for a long time. Also, what are you cheating on? If you're not on a diet, then you can't be cheating, because you're not breaking any rules, so it's the wrong word to use. By having a 'cheat meal' you're also not acting dishonestly or unfairly.

You're not doing anything bad by eating a pizza or a piece of cake. One single meal is not going to undo all the nutritional benefits of eating plenty of fruits and vegetables over the months/years. There's no such thing as a perfect diet, so eating foods you enjoy is simply a part of life. In fact, I would argue it should be encouraged! Eating for pleasure is so important for your health long term, and avoids the mentality of restriction or deprivation that sets you up for a binge-restrict cycle.

Some people also fall into the trap of scheduling a 'cheat meal' and then looking forward to it all week. This builds up the food to be something special and puts it on a pedestal. It makes it desirable to the point where exposure to that food is likely to send you into overdrive, where you feel you have to eat as much of it as you possibly can because this is your one chance to have it. But in reality, there's nothing that special about this food, and raising it so high above other foods simply makes it much more desirable: we always want what we tell ourselves we're not allowed to have. Take the food off a pedestal and it loses its power. It goes from being a 'cheat meal' to a particularly delicious and enjoyable meal.

Finally, if you call it a 'cheat meal', it'll likely take away from the enjoyment of eating it. Invoking the idea of cheating is automatically a negative association that implies you should feel guilty. And guilty is not how we want to feel after eating. Which leads me nicely on to the next term...

Guilt-free

Often, I hear the phrase 'guilt-free' being used to describe foods that are 'healthy alternatives'. Foods such as sweet potato brownies instead of ordinary ones, or cauliflower crust pizza instead of Domino's. These are recipes that are 'healthier' versions of so-called 'guilty pleasures' such as pizza, ice cream, chicken wings or cake.

What this is really saying is that the 'ordinary' version of these foods should make us feel guilty. If you buy a brownie that advertises itself as being 'guilt-free', does that mean the one next to it is full of guilt, and should therefore make you feel guilty? I think that's a horrible and sad way to look at food. It doesn't make us feel better; it just turns what should simply be enjoying a food you might have occasionally, but not every day, into a negative experience drenched with self-criticism.

Not only does that make us feel mentally miserable, it also increases the stress hormone cortisol, which makes you feel physically crap on top of that and potentially makes those cravings worse.

If you choose to eat a food that's maybe less nutrient-dense, or not traditionally seen as 'healthy', then you should be free to simply enjoy that food, and make that a deliberate choice for your own happiness. Feeling happy after eating something is not a crime. You don't need to do penance afterwards and compensate by eating only leaves for the rest of the day.

The term 'guilt-free' isn't just limited to food, of course. We now have guilt-free TV, shopping, desserts, drinks... Even the term 'guilty pleasure' is often used to describe our taste in music or television. It's a method of self-protection, as it pre-emptively shows disdain for our own choices before others can make fun of us. If we are unapologetic about enjoying something, we can be laughed at for it, and it can hurt us. Calling something a 'guilty pleasure' is self-deprecating and tells us we aren't allowed to do what we want because it's not right, normal or 'cool', or we haven't earned it.

Some might argue that guilt is a useful motivator to change behaviour and can aid self-control, but the research shows this isn't the case. In one study, people were asked if they associated chocolate cake more with guilt or celebration. The people who associated chocolate cake with guilt were not healthier or more motivated than those who associated it with celebration. In fact, they felt less in control around food and said they were more likely to overeat.[67] Guilt isn't helpful or a motivator. It leads to feelings of helplessness and lack of control, as well as self-criticism, all of which can encourage poor self-esteem and low mood.

In essence, no food should ever make you feel guilty.

All food is guilt-free.

Empty calories

Empty calories are supposed to be foods that contain large amounts of macronutrients (usually both fat and sugar), which provide calories, with a notable absence of micronutrients (vitamins and minerals) – so, energy-dense, nutrient-poor foods like doughnuts, soft drinks and alcohol.

The main problem with this is that we need calories to survive. Calories are the energy our bodies run on. We live in a food environment with more abundance than ever before, which naturally causes us to question and rebel against that which we have too much of (calories). But we can't just eat vitamins, minerals and phytonutrients to survive – we need calories.

Obviously I'm not saying go and eat as many of these foods as you want. But choosing foods purely based on how nutrient-dense they are completely ignores all the other aspects of eating, such as the social and cultural aspects, and the enjoyment of food. You don't have to avoid all 'empty calories' in order to be healthy, and only eat the most nutrient-dense foods you can find. Eating too many of these nutrient-poor foods (just like eating too much of anything) isn't recommended, but even calling them 'empty calories' reduces the enjoyment of them and encourages feelings of guilt and shame. As we've already established, these aren't helpful feelings when it comes to food. Enjoying these foods in moderation alongside plenty of fruits and vegetables is perfectly fine.

There's a notion that calories should always come with nutrients attached. 'Should' is a highly loaded and misleading word here. When we suggest that food should be a certain way, it implies that foods that aren't that way are somehow wrong, and therefore shouldn't be eaten. When we then crave these foods but believe they're wrong and bad, we try to turn to more nutrient-dense options that (at least in the vast majority of cases) just don't satisfy that craving.

In certain scenarios, these kinds of foods are exactly what someone needs. For example, someone undergoing chemotherapy may experience side effects such as nausea and vomiting. Weight loss during this process increases risk of mortality, so if all someone can stomach is pastries and sugary drinks, then that's what they should eat!

Calories are energy. Energy cannot be empty. Therefore calories are whole.

Good/healthy, bad/unhealthy

As humans, we love binary black-and-white thinking. So we like the idea of 'good' and 'bad' foods. We like dividing food up into these two neat categories. But food isn't 'good' or 'bad', it's just ... food.

The notion here is that eating 'good' foods should be encouraged, whereas eating 'bad' foods should be avoided. But the only food that is 'bad' for you is one that you're allergic to, or one that's gone off and mouldy. Any other food is inherently neutral. A food cannot be morally good or bad, regardless of the effects it may have on your health.

If you eat 'good' foods you don't become a good person, and when you eat 'bad' foods you don't become a bad person, but when we use this language that's what we're implying. 'I'm being GOOD today - I haven't eaten any chocolate', 'I really shouldn't eat this – I'm being so BAD'. No. The food you eat does not change your value as a human being, nor does it make you a better person than the one sitting next to you.

I don't use the word 'healthy' to describe food. There is really no such thing as a food that is intrinsically healthy, nor is there a food that is intrinsically unhealthy. Everything in nutrition is context-dependent and what may be healthy to one person is unhealthy to the next. Beans are celebrated in a vegan diet but shunned in the paleo community. A single food cannot impart health to an individual. It takes more than one food to be healthy, and it takes more than one food to be unhealthy. I believe you can have an overall healthy or unhealthy diet, but not healthy or unhealthy foods. Foods exist on a scale of nutrient density, and the order dramatically changes depending on what nutrient you are after. If you're calcium-deficient, then having some milk or leafy greens is arguably healthier than eating a carrot. If you're after omega-3, then oily fish is far healthier than eating a tomato.

'Healthy' is also often used to mean 'low-calorie', as if the two are somehow the same thing. Most of the arguments revolving around this say something along the lines of 'A food can be low-calorie but still full of artificial flavourings and nasty ingredients', which also isn't helpful at all – it's substituting one problematic language use for another. The equating of the two is linked to the idea that eating fewer calories is always better and weight loss is always the goal because thin equals healthy. By now it should be very clear that's not definitely the case. Multiple studies have also shown that when food items are labelled 'low-calorie' or 'low-fat' it adds a 'health halo' to these items, which means people are more likely to overeat on them.

I'd much rather people enjoy the exact food they want – not necessarily the lowest calorie version – and savour it without guilt.

I agree with using the term 'healthy' to describe an overall pattern of eating, but that property of healthfulness is not due to a single food, it's due to the overall picture, and that can easily include some less nutrient-dense and delicious foods like cake and chocolate.

Everything in nutrition is context-dependent, so based on that alone no food can be inherently healthy for everyone in every possible situation, nor can a food be inherently bad for everyone in every possible scenario. Even making assumptions and generalisations isn't ideal, as the very act of calling a food 'good' or 'bad' attaches moral values to it that don't belong there. Nutrition and food choice exist on a massive spectrum of grey shades and are almost never absolute.

Everyone has different nutritional needs and desires and preferences. A label of 'good' or 'bad' is far too simple and doesn't capture the complexity of our relationship with food.

Food can be nutritious, but not healthy. And all foods can be part of a healthy, balanced diet.

Junk food

There is no strict definition of junk food; the term used instead is High Fat, Sugar and Salt foods (HFSS). The legal definition is based on the UK Food Standards Agency (FSA) nutrient profiling of foods to determine what should and shouldn't feature in advertising to children.

The term 'junk food' is mainly used to describe cheap, mass-produced fast food. Anything artisan or 'wellness' is conveniently removed from this, even if the nutrient profile is essentially the same.

But what about 'wellness' brands? Your favourite energy balls, raw crackers and nut butters from health food shops are also mass-produced and made in factories. Yet because they're expensive and 'wellness' we wouldn't dream of calling these 'junk food'. The same bloggers who preach home-made food and eating as close to 'natural' as possible now either sell their own (factory-made) products, or are happy to promote them on their social media channels. Now obviously I'm not saying there's something wrong with eating these foods, but what really makes them different from non-wellness products other than marketing and cost? Is a burger by a wellness blogger automatically better or 'healthier' than one from McDonald's simply because it's more expensive?

Calling it 'junk' food is suggesting it's useless and a waste. It's a phrase that's used to cast a moral judgement on certain people's lives, and to signal our disapproval of that food, to label it as inferior. It's a way of shaming people for their food choices; by saying they're eating junk, the suggestion is they're treating their body like a bin and are therefore worthless.

Earn your food

As a human being, if you don't eat food, you will eventually die. Food is essential for survival. So why the hell should you have to earn something you need to survive? We are told that we need to 'earn' our food through exercise but never that we need to earn water, oxygen or anything else. Similarly, exercise is not punishment for having over-indulged. You can't negate or 'burn off' what you ate.

It's an interesting idea that people often believe – that behaviours or foods can cancel each other out in some way. But, of course, you can't turn back time, so all you can do is add foods or add movement – you can't take anything away.

Using food as a reward is something you were likely taught as a child, with parents probably saying something along the lines of 'If you finish all your homework on time you can have ice cream.' And while food can be a good motivator in some senses (it definitely encourages me to finish my work faster if I can feel myself getting hungry), motivation is very different from having to 'earn' food. Food should never be 'currency' that's earned by punishment.

If you feel like you overate and overindulged, that doesn't mean you have to punish yourself for having a good time. You can't change it, it's done, so the best thing you can do is simply move on. Do something positive and productive instead of battling with your body.

When you try to earn your food through restriction or doing exercise to burn calories, you are essentially saying you don't deserve it unless you engage in these behaviours, and you are defining your value based on food. That is not a healthy way to view food.

So, repeat after me: I am a human being and I ALWAYS deserve food because I need it to survive.

Fat-burning

We use metaphors of fire and burning to describe the eating process. Fire is both destructive and useful. It can get out of control and become greedy, leading to devastation and ruin, and it can also be the daily 'fuel' that keeps the human body alive and moving.

This idea of burning foods has partly come about because of the parallel to combustion engines in cars and how they burn fuel, and because of the use of bomb calorimeters to determine the calories in food for nutrition packaging.

Technically the body does 'burn' fuel, whether it's fat, carbohydrate, protein or alcohol. It converts the energy in the chemical bonds between the atoms in food into kinetic (movement) energy by breaking (metabolising) them. This process results in the formation of water and carbon dioxide.

The concept of 'You are what you eat' has led people to believe that fat outside the body must behave in the same way inside the body, which has translated into 'fat burning' and 'fat melting' food claims, and claims that you can literally melt fat and sweat it out. The fact is that the sweat is simply there to cool you down and has nothing to do with you metabolising fat. The carbon dioxide and water produced from fat metabolism are excreted by your body in the form of breathing and urine. Technically, you're breathing out and peeing out fat, not sweating it out. And even that is an oversimplification.

Despite all this, there is no such thing as a 'fat burning' food. Green tea, chilli, pepper, even celery ... all these have been touted as fat-burning. First, the idea that some foods require more energy for digestion than they give you is total nonsense.

You use approximately 10 per cent of your energy intake for digestion, so that still leaves 90 per cent left over regardless. Foods give you energy – they don't cause you to burn fat.

Second, while there is some evidence that shows your metabolism can be elevated slightly with the ingestion of certain foods, the effects on your metabolism are so brief and so minimal that they will not make any changes to your body composition, even in the long term. In comparison to moving your body – whether that's going for a run, going to the gym or just walking – the effect of foods on your metabolism is so small it's not even worth obsessing over.

Food metaphors are unavoidable, whether it's talking about human value or sex or femininity. Metaphors are an essential part of our cognitive processes. But what we can do is use these metaphors in a positive way, remove any negative ones from our vocabulary, and be more mindful of the language we use to describe food.

All these words and phrases are interlinked and have one big common factor: they moralise food and define your worth as a person by what you eat. Talking more positively about food and avoiding attaching morality to food is a simple way to improve your mental health and self-image.

Healthy language, healthy mindset, healthy life

WORD / PHRASE TO BANISH	REPLACEMENT	CONTEXT?
'Clean eating'	Balanced eating	'I haven't been eating well recently so I'm going to ~~eat clean~~ make sure my eating is more balanced from now on.'
'Real' food	Food	'I only eat ~~real~~ food.' 'Well duh, what else is there?'
Detox/cleanse	Healthier habits	'I drank so much alcohol last week I'm going ~~on a detox~~ to make sure I engage in healthier habits this week.'
Cheat meal	Indulgent meal	'I'm having a ~~cheat meal~~ indulgent meal this weekend and I cannot wait.'
Guilt-free	Delicious	'These brownies are totally ~~guilt-free~~ delicious.'
Empty calories	Less nutrient-dense food	'White bread ~~is just empty calories~~ may be a less nutrient-dense food but I'm really enjoying it.'
Good/healthy	More nutritious	'The salad may be the ~~good~~ more nutritious option on the menu.'
Bad/unhealthy	Less nutritious	'But I feel like having pizza even though it's ~~bad~~ less nutritious.'
Naughty	Listening to cravings	'Oh God, I'm ~~being so naughty~~ listening to my cravings by eating this chocolate.'

Junk food	Less nutritious food. Or, just call the food what it is.	'I'm craving ~~junk food~~ a burger tonight.'
'Earn your food'	Fuelling your body	'Time to hit the gym ~~so I can earn my food~~ then I'm going to fuel my body after.'
Fat-burning	Spicy/hot	(For this one, maybe just don't say anything.)

Using words like 'cheat', 'bad' and 'naughty' creates negative associations with food that we don't need. When we are in a place where we are feeling guilt or sadness at not being 'good' with our food choices, it takes away from the pleasure of eating and all the other wonderful aspects about food – whether it's celebration or togetherness or culture or nostalgia. It also creates a strong, restrictive mindset around food, providing space for rules, seeking perfection, failure and shame. This mindset leads you to think that you're eating something nutritious or 'healthy' because you feel you 'should' or you 'have to', which again takes away enjoyment, and also makes you want to 'cheat' even more. And so it creates a vicious cycle of 'being good', then 'cheating', then 'being good' again, and so on, which will only worsen as each cycle encourages further restriction and rules to try to prevent it happening again. Freeing yourself of these negative associations with food frees you from the cycle of rules and restrictions and stress and guilt, which is a much happier place to be.

5

ORTHOREXIA

'Perfectionism is a self-destructive and addictive belief system that fuels this primary thought: If I look perfect, and do everything perfectly, I can avoid or minimise the painful feelings of shame, judgement, and blame.'

BRENE BROWN

The pursuit of healthy eating is always seen as a good thing. But what happens when it gets taken too far?

Orthorexia nervosa is an obsession with healthy eating that's taken to the point where it is psychologically, socially and even physically damaging. It is still relatively unknown and misunderstood, but that's gradually starting to change. One of the biggest misconceptions about orthorexia is that it is simply a case of trying to be healthier, and what's wrong with that? Hopefully by the end of this chapter you'll understand why this condition is so much more than that, and why it's of growing concern.

The term 'orthorexia' is derived from the Greek 'ortho' ('correct') and 'orexis' (appetite). It was coined by the American physician Steven Bratman back in 1997 in response to a growing obsession with healthy eating that he noticed, particularly among yogis. Orthorexia is unusual in this respect, as the term first appeared outside scientific journals, and only gradually gained credibility among health professionals and scientists over time.

Orthorexia is characterised by an obsessive focus on healthy eating, food anxieties and non-medical dietary restrictions. It is not officially recognised as an eating disorder, but it has all the attributes of one.

The symptoms of orthorexia include making healthier food choices such as eating more fruits and vegetables, eating fewer refined white grains, and shopping in health food stores. It is also associated with other positive lifestyle habits such as exercise, not smoking and not binge-drinking. Individuals with orthorexia are also likely to share details about their way of eating and recommend it to friends and family.[68] This is one of the important differences between orthorexia and other eating disorders. One key characteristic of most eating disorders is that they are secretive and drive individuals to hide their thoughts and behaviours around food from the world. In orthorexia, the opposite seems to be true, and people are happy to be loud and proud about their dietary choices.

So far, all of these symptoms sound quite positive. But ortho-rexia is also associated with significant dietary restrictions, malnutrition and social isolation.

Currently, orthorexia does not appear in the Diagnostic and Statistical Manual of Mental Disorders (DSM)*, as official

---

* The DSM is the standard classification of mental health disorders used by professionals to diagnose mental health conditions.

diagnostic criteria are still being established and we still need more research to convince enough people that this is a real, distinct condition that deserves to be in the DSM.

The proposed diagnostic criteria for orthorexia include obsessive focus on healthy eating, food anxiety and dietary restrictions, with these behaviours causing clinical impairments.[69,70]

The primary criterion for orthorexia is an obsession with healthy eating or following a rigid dietary pattern in the pursuit of health. This can include the following ideas:

- Removal and avoidance of foods deemed to be 'unhealthy'. Dietary restrictions can be sudden, but usually escalate over time. Starts with elimination of specific foods, then entire food groups, and may lead to the point where someone is relying on 'cleanses' or fasts to 'purify' the body. These foods are removed without medical reason such as a diagnosed allergy or intolerance, and are not based on the instruction of a trained medical professional. Situations such as following a low FODMAP diet for IBS (under the guidance of a dietitian) or removing gluten from the diet following testing positive for coeliac disease would not fall under this, nor would removing pork from the diet for religious reasons.
- Worry about eating foods that are deemed 'unclean' or 'unhealthy', including worry about how this may affect the person's physical and mental health. In particular, worrying about increasing risk of disease, exacerbating disease, feeling 'dirty' or producing negative physical symptoms.
- Spending excessive amounts of time seeking out specific foods that are deemed 'safe', reading about food and health, and preparing these foods, including spending time weighing

out exact quantities of foods allowed. Also spending a large amount of money on these foods, which can include things like superfood powders or organic/biodynamic food.

* Feelings of guilt, shame and anxiety after consuming 'unclean' or 'unhealthy foods', often producing severe distress, and often with compensatory behaviours afterwards. For example, if someone eats a food they deem to be 'unhealthy' (accidently or deliberately), they may compensate by being more restrictive the next day, perhaps by doing a juice cleanse or cutting out another food.

* Intolerance of others' food beliefs, and a firm belief that their way is the best and only way to eat for health. The only exception to this might be someone who is following a similar dietary pattern, only slightly more restrictive. For example, someone who is mostly raw vegan might see someone who is 100 per cent raw vegan as even healthier and look up to their eating habits.

The second main criterion is that these preoccupations and obsessive ideas around food impair the person's health in some way. This is important, as it differentiates between someone passionately pursuing a healthier lifestyle and it becoming a clinical obsession. There is a scale ranging from disordered eating to fully clinical anorexia nervosa, and the same applies to orthorexia: there is a scale from simply picking up some obsessive ideas about food and having mild orthorexic tendencies to having more severe, clinical orthorexia. Diagnosis does require a cut-off somewhere on that scale.

In the case of orthorexia, these obsessions are clinical when the person's physical health or mental health suffers. Physical health can be affected because of nutritional deficiencies that can occur due to eating an unbalanced, restrictive diet, or unintended weight loss, again as a result of severe restriction of food groups. In orthorexia, weight loss is not deemed to be the primary goal, whereas pursuing health is. It can also be disruptive to someone's social life, affect academic or work performance as a result of the time spent thinking about food as well as potentially avoiding work situations involving food, and cause mental distress. This can especially be the case if body image and self-worth is mostly or totally dependent on compliance with what the person defines as 'healthy' eating behaviour. For me, one of the easiest ways to spot if someone has orthorexic tendencies or issues with food is by asking them how they would feel if their friends spontaneously asked them to go out for pizza tonight. If making this decision sparks anxiety, or a long and drawn-out thought process as to whether it's a good idea (ignoring any financial issues) and whether they can allow themselves to go, then their relationship with food isn't healthy.

Other traits that aren't considered to be essential to making a diagnosis but can also be helpful to identify can include obsessively focusing on planning food choices, buying food, preparing food and eating it. I've seen orthorexic clients who spend hours in a supermarket, obsessively checking the label on every single food item before discarding it. Food is often seen primarily as a source of health rather than a source of pleasure, and being near forbidden foods can be distressing, including watching others eat them. Body dissatisfaction doesn't tend to be centred around weight, but instead is focused on looking 'healthy' and 'well'. Even if their way of eating ends up leading to deficiencies and malnutrition, there is still a reluctance to give up this way of eating, instead focusing on what to eliminate next.

Case studies

Orthorexia is still quite new and unknown, and so I want to offer some examples of how it can manifest. Hopefully this will help increase your understanding of how it presents and how it differs from other eating disorders.

Client A was an overachiever who had a bit of a health scare and turned to Dr Google. They decided to cut out animal products from their diet, then when that didn't feel like enough they also removed gluten and 'refined sugar'. Over time this led to a fear of processed foods, so everything had to be made from scratch at home, including foods like hummus. They started doing the occasional juice cleanse to rid their body of any 'toxins' that might be contributing to their health. After a year of this they ended up in a situation where they had some vitamin deficiencies and severe anxiety about eating food that they hadn't prepared themselves, which meant they couldn't go out and enjoy a meal with friends, and their social life suffered. Their weight hadn't really changed significantly – the same clothes still fit – but they were miserable and so confused about what to eat.

Client B had a history of low self-esteem and poor body image, including being teased as a child. They joined a gym in order to fit more with the ideal body type, and decided to reduce their carbohydrate intake in order to speed up their progress. This was successful in the short term but then every time they went out and had a beer or ate a pizza with friends, they would feel bloated and wouldn't be able to perform well at the gym the next day.

Worried that this was hindering their progress, they decided to stop drinking, track their carbohydrate intake, and consume protein powders. They also stopped going out with friends. The result was some intentional weight gain, low mood, and anxiety around eating too many carbohydrates and not enough protein. Despite all this, their parents still commented that they looked 'weird and tired' the next time they saw them, which left them confused and disheartened that their routine wasn't working.

When client C's mother died of cancer, they became incredibly worried about whether they would end up getting it too. They started reading everything they could find about cancer, and were horrified at all the things they were told could cause it. Gradually, they started cutting out various foods, started scanning every food item for the ingredients list, and established food rules such as making sure to eat 10 different vegetables every day, with only one portion of each allowed to avoid repetition. All packaged foods were off limits, and they ended up with unintentional weight loss, vitamin deficiencies, and huge amounts of anxiety about eating anything that wasn't a vegetable, bean or pulse.

As you can see, in all three of these cases weight was not the focus, but health and avoiding disease was a common theme, as was anxiety. In this way, orthorexia can take up too much mind space with food and health, to the detriment of mental health and a social life.

Orthorexia and anorexia

The term 'orthorexia' was deliberately intended to have parallels with anorexia. The two definitely have some similarities.

Anorexia and orthorexia share characteristics such as perfectionism, anxiety, a need for control, and self-discipline. Both also share the negative feelings of guilt and anxiety when deviating from the set food 'rules'. However, while people with anorexia are preoccupied with the quantity of food, those with orthorexia are more concerned with the quality of food. The result of this in both groups can be elimination of food groups, which often leads to weight loss. But whereas with anorexia this weight loss is intentional and desired, with orthorexia weight is not the focus, and weight loss is not the ultimate goal. It is usually either not desired or comes secondary to the focus on health. As previously mentioned, one of the key differences is that those with anorexia tend to hide their eating habits, whereas those with orthorexia are happy to proclaim them to friends, family and even complete strangers on social media.

In addition to sharing traits with anorexia, there are also some similarities with obsessive compulsive disorder (OCD). These occur in the form of taking the time to carefully weigh and measure out portions of food, meal planning, and intrusive thoughts of food throughout the day, including away from meal times. The main difference is that in OCD, thoughts and obsessions are seen as being in conflict with the person's ideal self-image and cause distress to the sufferer, whereas the obsession with healthy eating in orthorexia is seen as normal, desirable even. Despite these similarities, orthorexia is still considered to be a separate condition, rather than a subtype of anorexia.

A common trend that's now being observed is that patients with anorexia are turning towards orthorexia during their recovery.[71] This may be a compromise by which patients continue to exercise control over their food intake, but in a more socially acceptable way. In patients with anorexia, those who have higher orthorexic symptoms seem to be closer to recovery. The orthorexic tendencies seem to allow them to feel more autonomous and able to learn to eat more 'normally', suggesting that orthorexic tendencies may be a coping strategy during recovery.[72] It's important to note, though, that I'm not saying those with orthorexic tendencies are recovered, as their eating behaviours are just as disordered as those of anorexic patients without orthorexia, which shows that the relationship with food isn't healthy and ideal.

Causes

Who is at risk of developing orthorexia? Current estimates suggest that it affects around 1 per cent of the general population,[73] similar to other eating disorders. But those especially at risk seem to be people who either have a keen interest in health and nutrition or are under pressure to look a certain way or be healthy for their job. This includes yoga instructors, dietitians, nutrition students, young athletes and exercise students.

Establishing the cause of any eating disorder is complicated, and orthorexia is no different. Trying to pinpoint an exact cause is difficult, as although there may be a clear trigger, it's likely there are also several underlying issues. Based on the research available (and there isn't that much) as well as my own experiences in my clinic, there are a few potential triggers and causes I've identified.

Feeling out of control

Similar to other eating disorders, control can play a big role in the development of orthorexia. If someone is experiencing difficulties in life that feel out of their control – whether it is parents going through a divorce, experiencing a break-up, abuse, or getting a scary diagnosis or a health scare (as with client A on pages 104–5) – food can be one thing that you can control. That level of control offers comfort and reassurance. It can manifest itself in the form of an eating disorder such as anorexia, or in trying to be the healthiest person you possibly can be, leading to orthorexia.

Societal ideals of beauty and health

Although orthorexia is not associated with a desire to be thin, the pursuit of health can still be a highly aesthetic goal, encouraged by a societal promotion of the 'thin ideal' or 'lean ideal' (see the example of client B on pages 104–5).[74] Ask someone what they imagine a 'healthy' person looks like and most likely they will describe a woman who is fairly thin (but not too thin), with curves but a fairly flat stomach, glossy hair and glowing skin. Basically, pretty much every famous wellness blogger. A 'healthy' man would be someone fairly lean, with visible muscles, smooth skin and a visible jawline.

Look at the *Love Island* contestants and this becomes blatantly obvious: everyone falls into these categories. They all fit the thin or lean ideal, which is why they're all considered to be attractive and desirable. If you haven't seen *Love Island* (either the UK or Australian versions), then think of shows like *The Bachelor* or *Are You The One* in the US. When someone doesn't fit these ideals, it's beyond understandable that this can lead to low self-esteem and body image issues.

The media is often blamed for eating disorders in general, but this is definitely an oversimplification that doesn't do the complexity of eating disorders justice. Societal ideals of beauty are linked to eating disorders through the images of beauty we see in the media, but whether an individual develops an eating disorder depends more on whether they internalise those images and compare themselves with the people who are shown as being beautiful. Because these images are often airbrushed and Photoshopped, the comparison doesn't end favourably and they feel like they don't match up to what they should look like. If someone sees these images and doesn't engage in this comparison, they are far less likely to develop an eating disorder.

In addition to pervasive beauty ideals, there has been an increasing moralisation of health, to the point where seeking good health is now seen as a moral obligation. By engaging in health behaviours (albeit to an extreme level), people are praised and seen as being good members of society, and not being a 'burden' on the healthcare system. Despite it being arguably quite selfish, it's seen as a selfless pursuit.

Low self-esteem

The feeling of not being good enough is a really horrible, unpleasant state that can lead to unhealthy coping mechanisms. Particularly among adolescents and young adults, there is enormous pressure to find a partner, fit in with peers, find a job and get accepted to a university, and the rejection that can follow is crushing to self-esteem. If you've been told (explicitly or implied) that you're not good enough, it's understandable that this can lead to eating issues, because one of the easiest and most obvious ways you can change is through your appearance (as client B did). Getting a 'revenge body' is now a commonly known phenomenon. The post-break-up haircut is even older. The idea of 'reinventing yourself' when you change jobs or go to university is focused almost purely on appearance. Making these changes is assumed to lead to improved self-esteem and self-confidence.

Individuals with orthorexia tend to be less satisfied with their bodies and have poor body image. There is a clear relationship between orthorexic symptoms and an unhealthy relationship with the body.[75] But changing your appearance to improve self-esteem is placing a plaster over the problem rather than addressing it directly.

Following a strict set of rules and being praised for following them, as well as receiving praise for trying to be healthier, only serves to increase the dependency of self-esteem on appearance and orthorexic tendencies.

Perfectionism

Low self-esteem and perfectionism are related, but I've listed them separately as I still feel they are distinct issues. While self-esteem is more about making up for perceived shortcomings by improving appearance, perfectionism is more about the need to be the best version possible in all aspects of life, including appearance. The pursuit of perfection is relentless and consuming, as perfection arguably doesn't exist. While you may be able to achieve 100 per cent in test scores, health and appearance is more nuanced, and can lead someone down the path of engaging in ever more extreme behaviours in order to achieve 'perfect' health.[74] Following a strict set of rules about what you can and cannot eat, to the letter and without any deviation, could be seen by the individual as a way of achieving perfection in this area.

Misinformation and fearmongering combined with health scares

A big trigger I often see in clinic is some sort of health scare, affecting either the individual or a close friend or family member. This health scare could be a parent being diagnosed with diabetes, a surprising blood test result, or suddenly experiencing severe bloating. What follows is usually a visit to Dr Google, where the ratio of accurate to inaccurate information is shocking at best. Overblown claims, fad diets and dubious bloggers with no health qualifications ... it's a minefield. For every ailment, there (almost definitely) exists a site on page one of Google that advocates elimination of certain foods or food groups. When an individual is in a vulnerable position, they are far more likely to accept these ideas about restriction and elimination of foods without questioning, which can set them down the path of orthorexia – particularly if the elimination helps them to feel better within a few days or weeks, as is often the case. Usually the foods suggested for elimination tend to be things like sugar, high-carbohydrate foods or processed foods, which tends to result in higher consumption of vegetables, an overall increase in nutrients and feeling healthier. There is also often a strong desire to feel better, because of the high cost involved, and that in itself can produce a placebo effect in the short term, before the increased restriction and anxiety leaves them feeling worse.

Dieting

Although the focus of orthorexia doesn't tend to be weight and weight loss, that doesn't mean that diets don't play a role. Diets may have gone a little out of fashion, but rather than disappear they have simply been rebranded as 'lifestyles'. Call it what you want, it's still a diet. The best example of this is 'clean eating'. The clean-eating movement is not a diet, it's a lifestyle, with a focus on health, although weight loss is usually offered as an added bonus. Clean eating has been hugely blamed in the media for the rise in orthorexia. I would argue it has been rightly demonised for the harm it has done, but it would be an oversimplification to suggest that it is the sole cause of orthorexia. The very use of the word 'clean' is an issue in itself (go back to Chapter 4 for a more detailed explanation of why the term itself is so hugely problematic), but it's the myriad of interpretations and variety of restrictions clean eating suggested that has made it particularly insidious, combined with its overwhelmingly successful use of social media. You could get into clean eating by removing all processed foods, then see another blogger tell you to avoid soy, so you do that too, then a number of posts show up that say how awful refined sugar is, so you also eliminate that. And so it goes on, until the list of acceptable foods is so small you end up with deficiencies and malnutrition.

When underlying issues such as low self-esteem or trigger events such as rejection or health scares are combined with the huge wealth of health misinformation online (particularly on social media), it provides the perfect storm for orthorexia to develop. By no means am I suggesting that social media is the cause of orthorexia, but having access to such volumes of information makes it far easier for orthorexia to develop and exacerbate.

Social media seems to be the biggest enabler of orthorexic tendencies. It's no coincidence that the whole 'clean eating' movement owes its success to social media such as Instagram – so much so that a dramatic link has been established between spending more than an hour a day looking at food and health accounts on Instagram and increased risk of developing orthorexia.[76]

Treatment

As orthorexia isn't currently in the DSM, there is no clear official treatment pathway in the same way that there is for other eating disorders. This also makes it much harder for people to access free treatment on the NHS, other than joining a long waiting list for counselling.

Based on my experience with orthorexia, as well as helping those who come to see me in clinic, the following pages list some of the methods I use to help improve people's relationship with food and themselves.

Re-education on nutrition

Often the ideas clients have about food are, through no fault of their own, based on misinformation. My clinic space is a complete no-judgement zone. Everyone falls for nutrition myths in life, and judging people for falling for misinformation is not helpful. What is helpful is understanding what ideas someone has about food and where those ideas have come from. Sometimes a client will be able to pinpoint the exact person on social media who scared them out of eating a food. Once these ideas and their origins have been established, we can begin to unravel these ideas and counter them with evidence-based advice.

The kinds of foods people are most likely to have misconceptions about are animal products (especially dairy), carbohydrates, sugar and increasingly more specific concerns such as soy products or lectins in beans.

Embedded within these ideas about specific foods is a general misunderstanding about what actually constitutes a healthy diet. The absolute black-and-white thinking around these foods and the imposed rules do not allow for any deviation. So sensible public health messages about reducing added sugar intake are translated into 'avoid added sugar' instead. Along with correcting false ideas about specific foods, there needs to be re-education on the importance of balance and moderation in eating, and the enjoyment of eating, instead of focusing on the tiny details. Moderation looks different for everyone, but in general it means eating a wide variety of foods without overeating any one in particular. It means eating lots of fruit and vegetables, but not feeling guilty about picking up a ready meal one day when you're coming home late from work and are too exhausted to cook. It means thinking about long-term patterns, not focusing on the details of every meal.

Food challenges

One of the first things I do with any client who has orthorexic tendencies is find out about their forbidden foods and food rules. This involves creating a list of foods considered 'forbidden' or 'unhealthy' as well as a list of 'allowed' or 'healthy' foods. In some cases it's also useful to create a list of foods that are sometimes 'allowed' but induce feelings of guilt, as this is a feeling we want to dissociate from food. In addition, we also create a list of food rules, which is particularly challenging, as many things won't feel like rules until you're asked to break them.

Once these lists have been created, I usually ask clients to rank foods according to the level of anxiety or guilt they produce: low-, medium- and high-anxiety foods. During every session we then discuss which food to tackle for their homework – usually starting with low-anxiety foods – and how best to go about this. I ask clients to make sure they are comfortable and relaxed before, enjoy the food slowly and savour it during, and afterwards think of three positive things about the experience. This is to help counter any negative thoughts around the food. Usually this results in one of two outcomes: either eating the food is a wonderful experience and they feel glad they could enjoy it, or they realise they actually don't enjoy that food as much as they thought, and it no longer has the same power as before. This process is slowly repeated with as many foods as needed, and it is always a collaborative decision. Later down the line we then tackle food in social situations that can be challenging, such as buffets, which seem to be anxiety-inducing for many people.

Social media 'cleanse'

A lot of misconceptions about food come from social media, particularly from Instagram. If, after going through a client's list of food anxieties, it appears that many of them come from bloggers and Instagrammers, I will take the time to go through their social media feeds with them. I'll identify potentially problematic individuals, ask them why they follow certain people and (most importantly) ask them how they feel after viewing the content they post. If they say they feel worse afterwards, I will hit the unfollow button for them. As someone who spends a lot of time on social media myself, I know how hard it can be to hit 'unfollow', as you feel bad for doing it, especially if you've been following someone for a while. So I do it for my clients to ease that process. Nine times out of ten they don't even notice that person is missing from their feed.

If someone spends a large amount of time on social media, particularly Instagram, then it can also be beneficial to actively try to reduce that time, at the very least to under an hour per day. I generally find that as I talk to a client about social media, after a while they realise themselves what a negative influence it can be and implement changes on their own, such as spending less time scrolling, or following more fluffy animals on Instagram – you can't feel bad about yourself while looking at pictures of cute puppies!

Improving body image and encouraging self-acceptance

I'm not a psychologist, so if someone has severe self-esteem and body-image issues, I will always recommend they see a psychologist or counsellor as well as seeing me. But improving people's relationship with food goes hand in hand with improving their relationship with themselves and their body, and working on both at the same time has a wonderful cumulative effect that's really encouraging for both me and them.

A lot of self-compassion and self-acceptance exercises can seem really awkward and hippyish, and that's a difficult hurdle for some people to overcome. But I have found them to be honestly helpful. When we engage in daily negative self-talk, those ideas about ourselves are constantly reinforced to the point where those thoughts can become automatic. Think about all the times you've looked at yourself in the mirror and automatically thought 'Ugh' or immediately picked up on something that's wrong with your reflection. To fight back against those automatic thoughts takes time and conscious effort. If you imagine an old-fashioned set of scales, like the Libra star sign, if you're adding negative thoughts daily to one side, your self-perception is massively skewed in the negative direction. It takes more than just one positive thought to counter all that; it takes continuously adding more and more positive thoughts to the other side of the scales before you even get to a point where you're in neutral. The point being that you won't magically wake up one day and fall in love with yourself – it takes work.

In order to counter negative thoughts, you first have to be aware of their existence, which is easier said than done when the thoughts are automatic. I'll usually start off by asking clients to make a note of every time they have a negative thought about their body, usually in the form of a tally (some people like to use emojis and code them according to the nature of the thought). Doing this over a couple of days will usually do the trick, and help make them aware of just how often they think negative thoughts about their body. Most of the time, people are shocked at how often they think these thoughts. It takes writing them down and seeing it visually represented to really appreciate this. That's the first step. After that, the next challenge is to counter each of the negative thoughts with something that's positive or neutral. Let's be honest, countering 'I hate my thighs' with 'I love my thighs' is pointless – you're not going to believe it. But countering it with 'My thighs allowed me to walk to work / do my workout / climb the stairs to my flat' is neutral yet far more effective. I arm my clients with a few examples and ask them to try this for a few days. It requires deliberate conscious effort at first, but the idea is that after a while the negative thoughts slowly become fewer and the positive/neutral ones feel more natural and believable.

As well as engaging in more positive self-talk, I also do self-compassion exercises with clients. Examples of this include making a list of 50 things you like about yourself (so hard to do), writing a letter to yourself as if you were a friend, or simply taking some time out in the day to consciously do something nice for yourself.

A lot of these techniques aren't just applicable to those with orthorexia; I see a great many people in clinic who are on the spectrum of disordered eating from years of failed dieting or reading fearmongering messages about food in the media, in books and on social media. If even one or two of these is helpful, then that's at least a great starting point.

Although there are some things you can do yourself to help with any orthorexic tendencies you may have, such as unfollowing people on social media and implementing some self-care practices, I would always recommend seeking out a health professional to guide you. The difficulty is that not many healthcare professionals have heard of orthorexia, let alone have experience in helping individuals who suffer from it. When people come to see me in clinic, it's usually because I'm the only person they know who recognises and understands what they're going through.

When seeking out a nutrition professional, look out for the letters RNutr, ANutr, or RD after their name. These letters are a sign that this person has studied nutrition at university as a science. Although there are many great nutritional therapists, I am always hesitant to recommend their services, as there is a very vocal and dangerous subgroup who promote pseudo-science, and so the title is no guarantee of evidence-based practice. With a registered nutritionist or dietitian, you can at least be sure they are held to a strict code of ethics. Many nutritionists or dietitians (myself included) offer people the chance to have a quick call before committing to a full session, just to ask any questions and see if they're the right person for you. If someone doesn't offer this, email them and ask what experience they have in orthorexia.

Quiz: Do you have orthorexic tendencies?

Please answer the following questions. If you have diagnosed food allergies or foods you avoid for medical reasons, don't include those in your decision-making. For example, if you have a peanut allergy but never avoid any other foods apart from peanuts, you might answer the question 'Do you avoid certain foods for health reasons?' with 'Never.'

	ALWAYS	OFTEN	SOMETIMES	NEVER
Do you avoid certain foods for health reasons?	4	3	2	1
Do you read nutrition labels?	4	3	2	1
Do you avoid foods with certain ingredients?	4	3	2	1
Are your food choices affected by worry about your health?	4	3	2	1
Is the nutritional value of food more important than the taste?	4	3	2	1
Do you have food rules?	4	3	2	1
Do you stick to your rules rigidly?	4	3	2	1
Do you think about food more than three hours a day? *	4	3	2	1
Do you seek out nutrition articles online?	4	3	2	1
Does eating healthy foods increase your self-esteem?	4	3	2	1

Do you spend a lot of money in health food shops?	4	3	2	1
Do you feel guilty about eating something unhealthy?	4	3	2	1
Do you find eating out in restaurants stressful?	4	3	2	1
Do you prefer to eat alone?	4	3	2	1
Have you recently cancelled dinner plans because you can't find anything for you on the menu?	4	3	2	1

* If you work in food, focus on food thoughts that aren't related to your work.

The usual tool used to assess risk of orthorexia in research uses language that isn't particularly user-friendly, so these questions are based on my own assessments I might use in clinic. Please note this is NOT a diagnostic tool, but can provide a guideline to see where your relationship with food is at.

- If you scored below 30: your relationship with food is most likely very good.
- If you scored between 31 and 45: You seem to have some anxieties around food, and it may be worth addressing these in case they become more severe over time.
- If you scored 45 or higher: You may be at risk of orthorexia, and I would recommend seeking professional guidance to help you get to a happier place with food.

6

FEARMONGERING FOOD

*'The only elimination diet most people should be
trying is one that eliminates myths and superstitions
about food.'*

ALAN LEVINOVITZ

If you want someone to avoid a food or follow a diet (cult),
then fear is the most effective tactic. Look at any diet book in
existence and they will use fearmongering tactics to push you
away from foods they deem 'bad' and in the direction of the
dietary dogma they are espousing, so they can sell you products
and plans and supplements.

Wellness uses phrases like 'Gluten is like sandpaper for the
gut' to scare you out of eating gluten, claims dairy is 'acidic'
and will cause cancer, and calls refined sugar 'toxic' while
encouraging you to eat the biochemically (almost) identical
coconut sugar.

Low-carbohydrate diet preachers use a fear of modern life and
an appeal to nature to claim that our modern high-carbohydrate

diets are killing us and that we need to eat the way our great-grandparents or distant ancestors did.

Almost every diet in existence instils a fear of processed foods.

Processed food

What is a processed food? Depends who you ask.

Refined and processed foods are deemed a moral and nutritional evil because they are low in fibre and therefore easy to digest. Because we are what we eat, the moral logic follows that if we eat 'lazy' foods it makes our bodies 'lazy', which will make us fat.

Our modern food system and processing has hugely improved the quality and safety of our food. There are fewer contaminations, fewer infections, and we can ensure better consistency in taste and so on. Having tinned and frozen foods also means preserving the nutrients in foods – frozen berries are just as nutrient-dense as fresh ones, but are cheaper and last longer, and tinned tomatoes are cooked for a longer shelf life, and the cooking means nutrients such as lycopene are more easily absorbed than in raw tomatoes. Processing also means that foods can be shipped around the world, enabling poor farmers to export foods and allowing our diets to be more diverse than ever before. Obviously, yes, it isn't all sunshine and rainbows, there are some downsides, and we should perhaps still be mindful that eating fresh berries in the middle of winter is special and not an everyday thing, but that doesn't negate the positives.

We like to divide foods into two neat categories: processed (bad) and unprocessed (good). Yet arguably almost all food is processed in some way. If you buy carrots already chopped they are processed, even if the ingredients are 100 per cent carrots. When you blend your fruit into a smoothie, that's a process; so is the extraction and purification of maple syrup and the freezing of peas. Whether you buy your hummus from Tesco or WholeFoods, it's still processed.

Equating 'processed' with 'unhealthy' is not quite accurate. One of the arguably healthiest things you consume on a daily basis is the most processed: water. The water that comes out of your tap is heavily processed to remove any harmful bacteria (to stop you getting dysentery), sediment and other impurities. If it wasn't processed, you'd be either dead or incredibly unwell right now from waterborne diseases. Water is probably the best example there is to show why processing isn't a bad thing.

Another good example is milk. Raw milk is milk from cows, sheep or goats that has not been pasteurised to kill harmful bacteria. It is seen in some subgroups to be healthier because it has not been processed. But pasteurisation is one of the greatest breakthroughs in food history. While raw milk can contain harmful bacteria such as *E. coli* and salmonella, and was blamed for one of the worst food-poisoning outbreaks in the UK in recent years, pasteurisation – the process of heating milk to 71.7°C for at least 15 seconds – kills off any harmful bacteria and makes milk safe to drink, as well as prolonging shelf life. But for those who enjoy raw milk, this isn't really the point; it's not just about the taste or the supposed health benefits, but about giving globalised mass production the middle finger and longing for a pre-industrialised past.

Beyond these specific examples are so many others I could have picked. Packets of ready-cooked grains, tinned beans, jars of pesto, dried pasta, even sliced bread. In the UK, it is a legal requirement for white flour to be fortified with iron and B vitamins, which means even the cheapest white bread provides you with these essential nutrients.

But we've now moved beyond simply having a dichotomy of 'processed' and 'unprocessed'; we also have the rise of the 'ultra-processed' foods. There is no current consistent definition of what amount of processing makes a food 'ultra-processed'. At what point does a food move from the 'processed' to 'ultra-processed' category? Because there's no consensus, it's often used to mean 'mass produced', 'factory-made', 'low cost' or 'low class'. It's certainly not 'posh' food.

But what about 'wellness' brands? Just like how with 'junk food' wellness brands are exempt, the same goes with 'ultra-processed' foods. Those energy balls technically count as ultra-processed too. Now obviously I'm not saying there's something wrong with eating these foods, but there's not really anything that makes them different from non-wellness products other than marketing and cost. The double standard seems unfair. Just because something is expensive it's seen as healthier and more desirable, when really there's no nutritional difference between a cheap flapjack with raisins and an organic, vegan, refined-sugar-free granola bar with goji berries.

The real issue with the processed vs unprocessed food dichotomy is that all foods lie on a continuous spectrum of processing, and the degree of processing is no guarantee of healthfulness. Even foods that fall into the 'ultra-processed' category, such as ready meals, can be highly nutritious and balanced.

Without food processing we would have been stuck in an era where food was far more dangerous, far more likely to give us disease, and where women would still be forced to spend large amounts of time cooking from scratch, rather than it being a choice. Yes, of course there are downsides to increased food processing, but the overall net effect on our health has, I would argue, been positive. We just take the benefits for granted now. And even the negative effects are from overconsumption of these foods, rather than the presence of the foods themselves.

Natural vs artificial

'Free from artificial colours and flavourings.'

We believe that natural is better than unnatural. But this way of thinking has two big flaws: first, 'What is natural?' is a really difficult question to answer. How do we define naturalness?

In dietary dogma, 'natural' appears to be an incredibly flexible term that is used as a proxy for acceptability across widely different diets. In veganism, drinking cow's milk is deemed unnatural as we are the only species to drink the milk of another animal. In the low-carb world, the process of refining carbohydrates is unnatural and therefore bad. In wellness, processed food that isn't as close as possible to how it's grown or harvested has been tampered with and is therefore to be avoided. In raw veganism, the act of cooking is deemed to be 'killing' vegetables and isn't how we're supposed to eat food. With so many conflicting ideas about what is natural and unnatural, how do we know who is right?

The answer is: no one is really right.

What almost all diets and diet books have in common is that they treat naturalness as the most desirable trait a food can have. Dieters should eat 'real' and natural foods, not artificial or processed foods (let's not forget that both artificial and processed are seen as the opposite of natural in the diet world). 'Good', 'healthy' and 'natural' foods are usually merged into one category and seen as interchangeable, and are contrasted with 'bad', 'unhealthy' and 'artificial' foods.

The black-and-white thinking of natural vs unnatural is the foundation on which the nutritional and moral logic of diets is built. It is manipulated to suit the needs of the diet.

Natural foods are seen as 'good' because they are pure and uncontaminated by any unknown substances used in processing. Marketing plays on this – how many times have you seen the word 'natural', e.g. 'full of natural goodness', 'only natural flavourings' and so on, and therefore been more convinced to buy it? Even if right now you're thinking you're immune to this kind of language, I challenge you to look in your cupboards or try to be consciously aware of it the next time you go food shopping.

But naturalness is complex and is misleading. Most diets also readily break their own rules about naturalness. For example, in low-carbohydrate diets, refined and processed foods are deemed unnatural and bad, but products such as cheese and processed meats are happily excluded from this. In wellness, processed foods are the unnatural enemies, yet superfood powders and other powdered supplements are deemed fine despite the processing required. Supplements often manage to worm their way into the approved 'natural' list, usually because they fix a deficit that is deemed unnatural and wrong.

Paradoxes like these are common in diets and discourses that focus on naturalness being the defining characteristic of health. For example, while white bread is often seen as processed and awful, wholewheat bread is given a free pass and deemed natural because it uses whole grains. But wholegrain bread is no more 'natural' than white bread, so it is arguably meaningless. In order to make wholewheat bread, manufacturers grind wheat into flour, mix it with water and yeast, and bake it at a high temperature. That is the bare minimum, as often other ingredients are added to improve shelf life (more on these later). The end loaf doesn't resemble the 'natural' grain of wheat in any way. Yes, you could make nutritional arguments for it being 'healthier' than white bread but it's still not really 'natural'. You could make the same argument for other foods such as tofu, almond milk, maple syrup or fruit squash. The point is that 'natural' here isn't really about how a food is produced or its ingredients; it's usually about the beliefs around how 'healthy' or 'acceptable' it is in a given diet plan. For low-carbohydrate diets, this means low-carb products are automatically good and 'whole', whereas high-carb products such as bread are 'processed'. In veganism, tofu and other soy products are 'good' and 'natural' for us to eat because they are plant-based, whereas a steak would be 'unnatural' and off limits.

The second flaw in this argument is that there are many 'natural' things that are not so good for us. The assumption that natural is always better and/or healthier is totally wrong. Organic products are deemed to be healthier because they use all-natural pesticides rather than artificial ones, despite there being no evidence that natural means less toxic. Some natural pesticides are more toxic than artificial ones, and some are less.

There is no clear relationship between naturalness and toxicity. There are so many natural things that can do you harm or kill you. Poisonous foods, foodborne diseases, allergic reactions... These are all totally natural things that care nothing for your well-being and are more than happy to lead to your demise.

Artificial flavourings are often chemically identical to the natural ones, and your body is unable to tell the difference. It doesn't have that kind of capability, and to assume it has is to romanticise the very complex yet indifferent process of digestion. Whether a flavour is natural or lab-made has no bearing on how healthy, safe or delicious it is. Flavourings made in a controlled laboratory setting have to undergo rigorous checks for quality control at every stage, and as such are often available as higher quality products than their 'natural' alternatives. Obtaining a flavouring from nature can also be difficult and expensive, as some products, such as vanilla, are rare. There is an argument to be made that artificial flavourings are therefore better for the environment.

In the end, there really is nothing 'natural' about the way we live and the food we eat. None of the foods now are remotely similar to how they used to be found in the wild. We have, over the course of hundreds or thousands of years, managed to selectively breed plants and animals to develop the characteristics we want. In particular, fewer seeds and sweeter flavours. Watermelons used to be all seeds and no flesh, but now we even have seedless grapes. My parents have always kept chickens, but when they grow old and die we don't eat them – they've been running around all their lives and the meat would be tough and not enjoyable like the chicken meat we're used to. I am typing this on a laptop, on a mass-produced IKEA desk and in a flat in a large city. There is arguably nothing natural about this at all. It's a strange irony that those who complain about unnatural foods tend to do so from their highly unnatural phones using a system of technology and electromagnetic signalling they can't explain. Simply put, pretty much everything that makes our lives cleaner, safer, longer and more comfortable is not natural.

The malleability of the word 'natural' has rendered it arguably useless. Calling a food natural is neither meaningful nor helpful, and can even mislead due to the moral baggage it carries. Instead, we should consider why these categories of 'natural' and 'unnatural' are being used. Is it to infer nutritional value or processing? Is it to further a political agenda? Is it to disgust or scare? These factors then need to be considered in their own right.

Only eat foods you can pronounce

There is something so wrong about this statement that has infiltrated its way into almost every dietary dogma. It's overly simplistic, and implies that your vocabulary and level of education should dictate your food choices, which isn't particularly scientifically sound. I would go so far as to say that using this statement is incredibly xenophobic and elitist.

Rather than using lack of knowledge as an invitation to learn about foods and ingredients, the user of this phrase implies that you are too stupid to understand and not worth justifying to. I think that's highly unfair. Blanket statements like this offer no nuance or opportunity for education.

It's also incredibly backward and anti-progress. Why should

we base whether or not to eat a food item simply on something as trivial as whether we can pronounce it? It invites a fear of the unknown, a fear of science and technology and innovation – all the things that have led us to this amazingly safe food system we have today. It's a classic fearmongering tactic, particularly as it's used to highlight 'OMG scary chemicals!'

I've said many times: everything is chemicals, and even something as harmless and loved as vitamin C can be 'scary' when you call it E300 instead. We are told by wellness only to eat foods you can pronounce, because anything with a scary name must be a scary unnatural thing. Never mind that scientists have a complex (yet highly logical) naming system for all identified chemical structures, so that something like omega-3 from fish oil can be called eicosapentaenoic acid ($C_{20}H_{30}O_2$), or vitamin B12 becomes methylcobalamin (or $C_{63}H_{91}CoN_{13}O_{14}P$), or vinegar is acetic acid (CH_3COOH). Not so scary after all, and definitely not something you have to avoid. On the other hand, I'll bet you can pronounce 'cyanide'; please don't eat it. I'll bet you can also pronounce 'poisonous mushroom', but again, please don't eat one.

Overall, this statement is yet another example of the elitist, middle-class, 'holier than thou' attitudes of the wellness and diet industries, which likely isn't helping the general population to eat healthier, only those who can afford to.

Nostalgia – don't eat the way your grandparents did

'Things were always better back then.' That's the narrative that almost every diet (or 'lifestyle') wants you to believe. It's a backlash against the rise of 'lifestyle' diseases and a distrust of the new, modern world, and so ties in perfectly with only eating foods you can pronounce. Whether it's looking back a few generations to 'eating how your grandparents did' or all the way back to the hunter-gatherer era, the implication is that we were healthier then compared with now.

Nostalgia is rife in low-carbohydrate diets as a yearning for periods of human history where surviving was a struggle, manual labour was the norm (both out hunting and in the kitchen) and the food system was less industrialised.

One of the main flaws in the argument of how we were healthier back then is that we now have far lower rates of communicable diseases, and this has extended our lifespan hugely. It sounds morbid, but in the end we have to die of something. Our ancestors didn't have high rates of cancer and heart disease because they mostly didn't live long enough for these kinds of diseases to develop. No food can do the incredible job that vaccines have done for our health.

'Don't eat anything your great-grandmother wouldn't recognise as food.' I doubt my great-grandmothers would have recognised kiwi, tofu, goji berries or 'paleo' bread. My great-grandparents were all white Europeans, so they wouldn't have recognised Indian or Thai or Mexican food either. If you happen to be Chinese, then your great-grandparents wouldn't recognise pizza, or if your great-grandmother was Italian she wouldn't recognise curry. We should be celebrating the fact that we are able to enjoy dishes from all over the world, and that we are able to find the ingredients to make dishes from our childhood or recreate something we ate on holiday based on a recipe we googled. Today's food is an incredible blend of local tradition, importation, innovation, technology and widespread availability. Our great-grandmothers cooked food for hours on end, whereas we have the privilege of being able to put it in a microwave or grill it in a fraction of the time.

Wellness is also massively hypocritical when it comes to this idea. We're told to avoid foods our great-grandparents wouldn't recognise, and in the next breath we're told how fermented foods like kimchi are the new trend, or how we should all be consuming this exotic superfood powder, or how adding turmeric to our latte makes it so much healthier. No white European great-grandparent would know about these foods, but somehow they're deemed to be ok?

Trendy superfoods in particular often have a notion of the exotic about them, but that alone doesn't make them appealing enough. The focus is always on the supposed health benefits, and this is given primary attention, with the historical and cultural narrative as more of an entertaining backstory that works well from a PR perspective. It's all well and good that apparently ancient civilisations were into their maca*, but it's only interesting to us if it can make us healthier too.

Matcha is a particularly interesting example here. While the cultural markers of other superfoods are woven into the narrative of how amazing they are, this hasn't been the case for matcha. It has been completely removed from its traditional preparation in Japan, and is now added to anything from smoothies to cakes

---

* If you're one of the few people who doesn't know what maca is, it's an expensive 'superfood' powder made from a Peruvian root, which companies grind up and sell to rich white people for lots of money. It's supposed to taste like caramel, but it actually tastes like dried clay.

and desserts. The reasons for its consumption are completely health-focused, with stories about its antioxidant content or alleged cancer-fighting properties, which effectively erases the cultural context from which matcha originates. In that sense, matcha has been reframed as a food from nowhere. What we've done is essentially food colonialism; we've taken something with strong cultural significance to others, and dominated and reshaped it to fit our wellness narrative of health above all else.

Ironically, even as people of colour are noticeably absent from the whole wellness and clean-eating movement, the movement's success depends on appropriating from non-white ethnicities. Foods like Medjool dates, turmeric, za'atar, quinoa and sweet potatoes have all been repackaged and commodified to the masses as part of wellness. And it's not just food; yoga is hugely whitewashed and reshaped into a fitness class, and Gwyneth Paltrow's Goop sells all kinds of crystals and 'chakra-balancing' products. These foods and practices would have once seemed weird and foreign, but because they're coming from white bloggers and celebrities who just pick and choose the bits of other cultures they like the sound of, they're now deemed worth listening to.

We want nostalgia, but we also want to appropriate other cultures at the same time, and wellness manages to balance the two perfectly in the name of health.

Contrary to this belief that our great-grandparents had it much better, we are actually eating much better than our great-grandparents, and we are likely going to live longer, healthier, easier lives than they did. I think our great-grandparents would be excited to know about all the new and interesting foods we have available, and how easy it is to achieve a varied diet.

Most people, if you ask them, will say things were better when they were younger and that the world is getting worse. We have a tendency to romanticise the past because our memory is more likely to forget about the bad events in our past and instead is prone to dwell on the good things. We take for granted the things we like that improve our lives such as smartphones and cheaper air travel, and focus on the negatives that we feel have made our lives worse. In general, people just don't like change.

Nostalgia is so powerful because it is contrasted directly with the idea that anything modern is bad and out to get us. It creates a beautiful dichotomy of modern equals evil and past equals good. Our modern food system is portrayed as a disaster with its processed food and widespread availability. Yet as modern food became more available, populations grew taller and stronger, and lived longer. People didn't have to spend so many hours slaving away in the kitchen, and diets became more varied, with a far lower chance of starvation. Going from the general to the highly specific, our modern food supply has allowed us to fortify foods with extra vitamins to prevent deficiency, and allowed us to create machines that do a far more efficient job at kneading dough or grinding cocoa beans.

Toxicity discourse and sugar

If you want to induce fear about a specific food, then claiming that it's toxic is one of the easiest ways to achieve this. In recent years, this is exactly what we've seen with sugar.

But comparing new foods, and specific foods like sugar, to addictive drugs is nothing new or unique to any particular dietary dogma. In the 1960s and 1970s there was intense wide-spread fear of sugar, and recently it's reared its ugly head again.

This is so successful because it allows accurate (and boring) public health messages aimed at reducing consumption to become inaccurate and sensationalist messages of avoidance. So instead of public health advice to reduce free sugars to less than 5 per cent of daily energy intake, we see advice to go on a 'sugar detox' and how to cut this 'toxic' substance out of our lives. No one wants to eat something they know is toxic – because toxic implies that it's dangerous at any amount, not just large amounts.

That's just not true. As any chemist will tell you: the dose makes the poison. Toxicity is dependent on quantity, and anything in food can be toxic at the right level. Some examples:

- Drinking more than 100 cups of coffee in quick succession could kill you.
- Eating more than 50 bananas in one day could give you potassium poisoning.
- Chewing the seeds of 20 apples one after the other could give you a lethal dose of cyanide.
- Eating 4–5 raw kidney beans would start producing horrible symptoms, and eating around 300 g per kilogram of body weight could kill you.
- Drinking more than 6.5 litres of water in a short space of time can kill you. This has happened to some marathon runners after they've crossed the finish line.

These are all perfectly natural products, but as we've seen, nature doesn't really care if you live or die.

Sugar is an interesting case as all healthcare professionals can agree that eating too much of it is not a good thing, yet fearmongering narratives around sugar have existed for a long time, way before the increase in type 2 diabetes and the so-called 'obesity epidemic' that has fuelled the modern anti-sugar crusade. In the nineteenth century the anti-sugar brigade blamed a whole host of conditions on sugar, such as indigestion and increased sexual desire. Eating sugary foods like chocolate and ice cream became associated with women in particular, and the inability to 'resist temptation'. Fast-forward and replace indigestion and sexual desire with obesity and type 2 diabetes and not much has really changed.

Many people think that a diet completely free from sugar is far healthier than a diet that contains just a little sugar, despite no evidence to suggest this is the case. This idea does make sense, however, if you compare sugar to illegal drugs. One line of cocaine probably won't kill you, but it can be addictive, therefore even a little cocaine is dangerous. Therefore if sugar is also considered addictive, then even a little sugar could be dangerous too. Both also conveniently happen to be white powders, making the comparison even easier for fearmongers. The fact that leading researchers in the field of addiction say there isn't enough evidence to suggest sugar is addictive, and that calling it addictive isn't helpful on a public health level,[77] is irrelevant and holds little power in the face of scaremongering.

The nocebo effect

Fearmongering tactics are so powerful that they can produce

physical symptoms in people, despite a complete lack of allergy or any real issue with a food. This is the nocebo effect, and shows just how incredible the mind can be.

We are all familiar with the placebo effect, whereby improvements in symptoms can occur even without any medical intervention. Give someone a sugar pill and tell them it's a painkiller and it's likely that their headache will improve. Place someone on the operating table, cut them open and sew them immediately back up again and they'll report feeling better afterwards, despite a lack of actual surgery taking place. Of course, this doesn't work 100 per cent of the time, but it works far more often than can be attributed to chance.

While placebo has positive effects, nocebo is negative. Give someone a sugar pill and a list of side effects and there's a chance they'll report experiencing some of those side effects. In food, this can occur with a wide variety of foods, including lactose and gluten. When people who claimed to be gluten sensitive were fed a diet they thought contained gluten, they reported symptoms even though there actually wasn't any gluten in the food.[78] Similarly, when people who are lactose intolerant are given a sugar pill, some experience symptoms such as abdominal pain.[79] To say this is 'all in the mind' is true, and in my eyes doesn't dismiss these effects but just shows how dangerous fearmongering tactics can be. If someone has become convinced that a certain food will do them harm, then not only does it have psychological implications but these can manifest as physical symptoms that are painful and cause distress. Fearmongering makes it harder to distinguish who is actually allergic or intolerant to a food and who is experiencing a nocebo effect due to the misinformation they've been fed. The solution is not to eliminate the foods that are the source of anxiety, but to eliminate the myths and correct the misinformation around these foods that are responsible for inducing that anxiety in the first place – which is hard, considering a new diet guru spreading fear appears every day.

Food and cancer scares

Cancer is probably the disease that instils the most fear in people, more so than type 2 diabetes or heart disease or dementia. With the statistic that one in three people will be diagnosed with it, it's hardly surprising. Everyone has been affected by cancer in their life, either directly or indirectly. This has made it especially vulnerable to fearmongering.

As such, there are many misconceptions about cancer. When researchers surveyed the public they found that people's ideas about what causes cancer were wildly inaccurate.[80] Forty per cent of people wrongly thought that stress and food additives caused cancer, 33 per cent incorrectly believed that electromagnetic frequencies and eating genetically modified foods were risk factors, 19 per cent thought microwave ovens and 15 per cent said drinking from plastic bottles. This is all despite a lack of scientific evidence for any of these.

The main problem with these beliefs is that they can make people fearful and anxious about the food choices they make, particularly when it's something they feel is out of their control. By improving the accuracy of people's beliefs about what causes cancer, we might be able to reduce people's fear and anxiety, while also helping them feel more empowered about their ability to reduce their risk.

When researchers chose 50 common ingredients from a cookbook, they found that 80 per cent of them had research that showed an increased risk of cancer, although the evidence was mostly weak.[81] These kinds of studies are the basis for the headlines we see on a regular basis that shout 'X food causes cancer', even though they have only found an association (and a weak one at that), and a single study is not enough to determine this for sure – we need to look at the overall picture of many studies in order to establish this. Essentially, when you read these headlines, they're probably not really worth taking notice of.

The big fearmongering around cancer that's become mainstream recently focuses on animal products, specifically dairy. People are trying to extend moral and ethical concerns around specific foods to nutritional concerns. There is an assumption that because a food is bad for the environment or for animal ethics, it must therefore also be bad for humans, because we like to think of food as black and white, 'good' and 'bad', and if a food is 'bad' in one sense it must therefore be bad in all senses. But food doesn't work that way. As a result, there are some really awful myths about dairy floating around the Internet.

Dairy is a very broad food group, and within that we have evidence of health benefits for cheese, yogurt and whole milk, and that dairy products are associated with a reduced risk of several cancers, including breast cancer. Also, both whole and low-fat milk consumption is associated with lower risk of heart disease and type 2 diabetes.[82] The fearmongering about hormones in milk causing cancer just doesn't stand up to scrutiny.

The Internet is unfortunately probably the worst place to seek advice and recommendations on cancer. An article examining alternative cancer cures on the Internet found the quality of information given 'had the potential to harm cancer patients if the advice provided was followed', and even sometimes actively discouraged patients from seeking effective conventional treatments such as chemotherapy.[83] This is serious, considering that those who deviate from conventional cancer treatment are 2.5 times more likely to die within five years.[84]

Carbphobia

Carbohydrates feature as the backbone of almost every great civilisation. Look around the world and carbohydrates are and were the staple pretty much wherever humans gathered in large numbers. We may hark back to hunter-gatherer times, but every year our most accurate interpretation of when we first started eating carbohydrates and making bread goes back earlier and earlier. We domesticated wheat, and it in turn domesticated us, and we settled where it grew. All over the world humans thrive because of wheat, rice and maize. Yet we're going through a low-carbohydrate craze right now, and carbphobia has become a serious issue.

Even excluding hunter-gatherer days, low-carbohydrate diets go way back to Greek Olympic athletes who consumed high-meat, low-carbohydrate diets. In the 1920s the ketogenic diet (which we'll come back to) was first used to treat epilepsy in children, with great success. Since then, every five to ten years there's been a surge in popularity of low-carbohydrate dieting, whether it's the Inuit diet, Atkins, the Paleo diet, the South Beach diet and, returning to present day, the ketogenic diet for the general population – a diet so low in carbohydrates it causes the body to enter a form of starvation mode.

Like any diet, low-carb high-fat (LCHF) diets claim to have the best answer for weight loss. But it goes beyond that, with drastic claims about reversing diabetes, treating any number of health conditions, how current dietary guidelines are killing us, and how we should avoid carbs and instead eat as much saturated fat as we want. Let's examine some of these claims.

The idea that LCHF diets are uniquely the best way to lose weight doesn't stand up to scrutiny. Randomised control trials (RCTs) are rare in nutrition, as it's hard to force people to eat one way or another, especially in the real world and not in a controlled laboratory setting. But RCTs on low-fat vs low-carb diets show there is no real difference between the two.[85] And, as we saw a few chapters back, both are equally ineffective in the long term on a population level.

Because of results such as these, we also know that LCHF isn't uniquely positioned to treat or reverse type 2 diabetes. In some cases it absolutely does help, but equally so can things like getting adequate sleep, stress management, eating a Mediterranean diet or increasing exercise. The idea that LCHF is a special cure for diabetes is linked to the idea that carbohydrates cause diabetes. It's quite easy to see where this idea has come from, as eating carbohydrates causes the hormone insulin to be released in the body, and type 2 diabetes is characterised by a resistance to insulin as well as very high blood sugar levels (if you need a reminder, go back to the emotional eating chapter section on hormones). But nothing in nutrition is really that straightforward, and this carbohydrate-insulin model has been debunked as overly simplistic.[86]

Also, the rise in consumption of grains and higher carbo-hydrate diets precedes any dramatic rise in 'lifestyle' diseases by a few hundred years. To suggest that carbohydrate consumption is the root of these problems firstly undermines the complexity of the human condition and secondly fails to account for this time period where we were eating plenty of grains yet were allegedly totally fine and healthy.

But it's not just the fact that they're misunderstanding the science of saturated fats and carbohydrates that's damaging to our health; it's the excessive fearmongering around carbo-hydrates and the bullying of those who dare to disagree with them that has led me to focus my attention on this group. In my clinic and online, carbphobia is the most common thing I see. Anyone with any food issues or disordered eating who comes my way has some issues with carbohydrates. They feel the need to plan meals without grains, do carb-cycling, or avoid grains and sugars altogether. They feel that if they don't do these things they will gain weight, develop diabetes or make themselves unhealthy in some way.

We have significant and overwhelming evidence to suggest that eating whole grains, beans, fruit and vegetables comes with some serious health benefits. What the LCHF movement does is essentially place all these foods in one category together with sugary breakfast cereals, energy drinks and so on. All these carbohydrate sources are being lumped together, and we're told they're all bad and all equivalent to X teaspoons of sugar. This is such a ridiculously reductionist approach, as foods like wheat, for example, contain fats, proteins and micronutrients in addition to carbohydrates. On top of that, we don't tend to eat foods in isolation, we eat them as part of meals, and the combination of foods in a meal affects digestion and how quickly we absorb nutrients. This comparison is biochemically non-sensical, as sugar (sucrose) behaves very differently from long, complex chains of glucose molecules joined together. To suggest they are equivalent in some way is purely intended to scare.

Blaming the UK dietary guidelines for an increase in type 2 diabetes and other health issues doesn't exactly make sense. Why? Because people don't follow them. You can't blame the guidelines if people aren't adhering to them. In fact, research shows that if we did adhere to dietary guidelines, we'd be better off as a population. There was a study in 2015 in which subjects were told either to follow a diet pattern that adhered to the dietary guidelines or to follow a typical British diet* (the control group). After 12 weeks, the dietary guidelines group were eating more fibre and more unsaturated fats, lower added sugars and saturated fats, but the same amount of total fats as the control group. They also ate around double the amount of whole grains. When the effects on heart-disease risk factors were assessed, the researchers found that the dietary guidelines group were predicted to have a 15 per cent lower risk of developing heart disease, as they had lower inflammation, reduced blood pressure and lower LDL ('bad') cholesterol.[87] This is because the guidelines state to increase vegetable consumption, increase whole grains, increase fibre, and reduce both saturated fat *and added sugar* – the latter of which conveniently gets forgotten in LCHF narratives. Yes, the guidelines used to recommend reducing total fat intake, but that's definitely not the case any more.

---

* A typical British diet is a pessimistic affair: low in fibre, not enough vegetables, high in added sugars, and low in oily fish.

LCHF advocates argue that previous guidelines on cholesterol and fats were incorrect, and we're all getting sicker, therefore we need a different approach, and the answer is low-carb. They couldn't be more wrong.

We now know that reducing total fat isn't necessarily the answer on a population level, but it's the types of fats we're eating that matters. Eating sources of unsaturated fats such as oily fish, plant oils like olive oil, nuts, seeds and avocado is highly beneficial. But what any healthy diet pattern has in common – whether it's relatively high-fat like the Mediterranean diet, or more low-fat – is that it is low in saturated fats. The government recommendations have changed their stance on total fat because the science has become better, but the recommendation to maintain a low intake of saturated fat still stands because the research supports it.[88]

The science is so beautifully nuanced now that we're looking not just at individual nutrients but at individual foods, so we know dairy foods such as cheese, milk and yogurt, despite technically being good sources of saturated fat, don't have the same negative effects on health and actually carry a whole host of benefits.[82] That same nuance has been applied to whole grains and found them to be highly beneficial, and not something to be afraid of.[89]

It would be unfair to suggest that low-carbohydrate diets are *always* bad and unhealthy, and that would make me no better than the leaders of the low-carb movement. The fact is that sometimes a low-carb diet is what works well for someone and makes them feel good. The health benefits of low-carbohydrate diets have little to do with the fact that they're low-carb – they depend almost entirely on what those carbohydrates are replaced with. The research suggests that if they are replaced with higher amounts of saturated fat, then the effects on health and mortality are detrimental; whereas a low-carbohydrate diet that includes some beans or pulses, is high in fibre and lower in saturated fat has similar health benefits to the Mediterranean way of eating, and offers no increased risk of mortality.[90] So, once again, it comes down to overall dietary pattern rather than the inclusion or exclusion of particular foods. But this still does not absolve the low-carb movement of any responsibility, as many leaders in that area still claim you can eat as much saturated fat as you want without causing yourself any harm. This is categorically wrong and harmful.

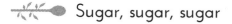 ## Sugar, sugar, sugar

Sugar is the perfect example to illustrate how all these fear-mongering tactics come together:

- Processed vs unprocessed: Refined sugars are so processed and therefore deemed bad for us, whereas unrefined sugars (despite also being processed) are apparently good and healthy things.
- Natural vs artificial: Refined sugar is deemed to be 'bad', whereas honey is frequently cited as being healthy due to the fact it's deemed to be more natural. Also, sugar is seen as toxic, unless it's naturally occurring in fruit, in which case it's totally harmless.
- Only eat foods you can pronounce: Fearmongers state how sugar has many names on food packaging and look at how scary and unnatural some of them sound.

- Nostalgia: Many years ago we didn't eat sugar and we were so much healthier back in those days (not true), then this strange exotic ingredient came to our shores and wreaked havoc on our health.
- Toxicity: Sugar is deemed toxic and is compared to illegal drugs.
- Nocebo: If you're told enough times that sugar is addictive and can cause massive mood swings, that can manifest in the form of headaches, shakes, and a compulsion to eat sugary foods.
- Cancer: There is a pervasive myth that sugar 'feeds' cancer cells, even though technically sugar 'feeds' all cells – glucose is the fuel that can be used by every single cell in the body. There's no way you can tell your body that the food you eat (which generally converts to glucose) should only feed healthy cells, not cancer cells. You just can't do that. Also, cancer is far more complicated than this, and to suggest otherwise is an insult to any person who has developed cancer – you're implying it's their fault because they ate sugar. That makes you an awful human being.
- Carbphobia: Sugar falls under the carbohydrate umbrella, therefore it's causing all our modern problems, allegedly.

These fearmongering ideas about food have spread primarily due to the media and social media, including new avenues such as Netflix, where we have huge amounts of information at our finger-tips. The next chapter will explore these mediums a bit further to see their effects (both positive and negative) on our health.

Fearmongering Quiz

Next time you read or watch something related to nutrition and health, watch out for these warning signs:

	YES	NO
Clear good/bad foods		
Labelling a food or ingredient as toxic without describing the dose		
Something is deemed bad because it's unnatural		
Something is deemed good because it is natural		
Assuming something is bad because you don't understand it		
Assuming something is bad because it's new or foreign		
Assuming something is good because it's been done many times before		
Talk of 'good old days'		
Modernity and technology as the enemy		
Claims that you are addicted to a food		
Claims of a food or ingredient causing disease		
Selling of a simple answer to all problems		
Most importantly... do you feel knowledgeable or stressed/scared/anxious afterwards?		

7

SOCIAL MEDIA, MEDIA AND NETFLIX

'Don't compare your behind-the-scenes with somebody else's highlight reel.'

STEVE FURTICK

In 1995, American researcher Robert Kraut and colleagues provided Internet access and a computer to 93 households that had previously had no Internet experience at all, and tracked their psychological health over several years.[91] After one year of using the Internet, the researchers concluded that greater Internet usage was linked to more signs of depression and loneliness. Although several years later they found that most of the negative impact had dissipated with time, since then the general concern over the impact of technology (and particularly the Internet) on health has escalated.

Now technology is more than just about Internet access and television. It also includes social media, which we have access to 24/7 from our phones, it's about Netflix and access to a greater variety of videos than ever before, and it's about the continuing impact of the images and bodies we see all around us, reinforcing the idea that there is one ideal body shape, one ideal diet, one way to be healthy.

These influences have existed for an arguably very short period of human history, and arguably during that time they have had a huge impact on the way we live our lives. Try to imagine a life without television, magazines, newspapers, the Internet, social media or advertisements. Some might consider this to be paradise, whereas to others the idea is horrifying.

Social media

As of 2018, Instagram now has 1 billion monthly active users, Facebook 2.23 billion and Twitter 335 million. In 2017, there were almost 2.5 billion people using social media, with over 70 per cent of Internet users having an active social media profile. At the time of writing there are almost 3 billion social media users around the globe. That's a lot of people.

Almost everyone in developed countries has at least one social media profile, with many people having several. We spend hours and hours online on these platforms, especially the apps, and each notification lights up our phones demanding our immediate attention. I'm going to assume that if you're reading this, you're probably well aware of the different social media platforms and what they look like.

But what impact do these sites have on our health? It doesn't look too good.

Depression and anxiety

Major depression is more than just feeling a bit down. It's a serious health issue that affects tens of millions of people each year, yet only a fraction of people receive adequate treatment for it.

Using social media has been linked to increased depression in young people. In one interesting study, those who spent the most time per day on social media had a much higher risk of depression than those who spent the least time online.[92] More frequent Instagram use has been shown to have a direct association with greater levels of depressive symptoms.[93] There doesn't seem to be a popular social media platform that hasn't been linked with depression in some way.

Interestingly, on Twitter, researchers have used tweet patterns to detect the onset of depression in individuals. They detect this through measuring lower social activity, greater signs of negativity, high focus on the self rather than others, increased voiced concerns about relationships, and being more likely to express religious thoughts.[94] There is the hope that, in the future, Twitter may be a tool by which undiagnosed individuals may be alerted to their altered behaviour in the hope they can seek help earlier.

Unlike other uses of the Internet, social media involves receiving notifications and alerts at all times of the day. These constant notifications create pressure to be constantly available and contribute to a severe case of FOMO (fear of missing out). This helps explain why social media use is linked to increased anxiety,[95] particularly among young adults, and has led to the term 'social media anxiety disorder' being coined, where people feel stressed and anxious if they are not able to check their accounts and notifications regularly. Receiving and seeing a notification provides a small dopamine hit, which makes you feel good, and while I wouldn't necessarily go so far as to say it's addictive, it can leave you feeling disappointed if you check your phone to see no notifications at all. In some cases, for some people, this can lead to an endless feedback loop with a need to post more and receive more likes in order to feel just as good as they did initially.

The symptoms of social-media anxiety are not set in stone and are variable (see the end of this chapter for a rundown), but in general they tend to involve an obsessive need to maintain an online reputation or persona, while also ensuring that popularity is maintained, and communication is active and regular. A little bit of this kind of behaviour is arguably normal and healthy – it makes sense to care what others think of us in our social society – but when it starts to interfere with normal daily functioning, and when it starts to inhibit face-to-face social behaviour, then it may be problematic.

Eating issues and social media

Eating disorders and related behaviours have been linked with social media use. Viewing health- and fitness-related content on social media means you're more likely to have an eating disorder, but also more likely to engage in healthier behaviours such as not binge-drinking or using illegal drugs.[96] Spending more time on social media in general (rather than a specific site) is also linked to greater odds of having eating concerns.[97]

In people who already have an eating disorder such as

anorexia nervosa, a high level of Facebook use is associated with greater levels of symptoms,[98] and viewing pro-anorexia websites and forums have greater negative effects[99] compared with people who don't view these sites.

There is a strong 'image first, text second' rule on Instagram, which allows for easy comparison of bodies, particularly bodies that fit the thin or lean ideal. Instagram tends to reward bodies that fit this ideal, as they get more likes and engagement. High social media usage in general is linked to increased body image concerns and disordered eating behaviour.[100]

Around a quarter of young people turn to social media to find information about healthy eating, which is concerning considering that pretty much all Insta-celebs or people with large followings have no relevant qualifications and definitely aren't experts on nutrition. The advice given online is generally misleading and isn't regulated in the same way that health claims in advertising are. So it's no wonder that many people believe that exclusion of food groups is important for health, and that people fall for crazy diets peddled by people they follow and look up to.

The entire 'clean eating' movement owes its success to Instagram. The pioneers of this movement relied heavily on this platform, and had (have, in some cases) a powerful presence, reaching and influencing millions of people, despite having no formal qualifications in nutrition or cooking. Due to Instagram being an image-based platform, it may be that people are more likely to follow advice or imitate the diets of Instagram 'celebrities' such as these, as they feel a more personal connection than they otherwise would with a text-based platform. As such, Instagram plays a key role in the development and maintenance of disordered eating patterns associated with orthorexia nervosa, to the point where high Instagram use is a risk factor for orthorexic symptoms.[76] Even though most of these bloggers have now distanced themselves from the term 'clean eating', there still exists a large body of fearmongering, misleading information on Instagram, which can trigger and reinforce orthorexic ideas.

Self-esteem and social comparison

Social media and self-esteem are tightly intertwined. Positive feedback on your profile seems to enhance social self-esteem and well-being, whereas negative feedback seems to decrease self-esteem and well-being.[101] In contrast, viewing your own profile appears to increase self-esteem.[102] It seems that the more emotionally invested you are in your social media accounts and profiles, the more they affect your self-esteem, so people who feel a strong emotional connection to social media are most at risk.

The negative impact of social media on self-esteem seems to be mediated by social comparison. Social comparison is the tendency to compare yourself with others on specific attributes, and we are more likely to compare ourselves with someone we think is similar to ourselves – our peers.

Evolutionarily, throughout history we have compared ourselves with a small number of people within our social environment, i.e. people within our tribe or small social circle. The rise of social media has drastically shifted who we consider our peers and who we therefore compare ourselves with. Our ancient brain hasn't had time to adapt to this new social environment, which has only been around for the last 10 years or so (Instagram launched in 2008).

The prefrontal cortex in our brains is most associated with higher cognitive functions such as critical thinking, and is moulded by our environment up until the age of around 25. Now that almost every young person is on social media, and follows a variety of people, including friends, celebrities and influencers, the Instagram feed is interpreted as reality and helps shape this social comparison. This means the brain can't tell the difference between your neighbour or an Instagram model, and they are interpreted as peers of the same social group and therefore a reasonable target for comparison. Naturally, this doesn't bode well.

People are far more likely to make upward social comparisons on social media compared with real life. Upward social comparisons are when we compare ourselves with other people who we perceive as being slightly better than us or who we look up to in terms of certain characteristics, whether it's appearance, fitness or academic grades. For example, although you likely won't compare yourself to Albert Einstein, you will compare your grades with those of others in your class, especially those who you perceive to be on a similar or slightly higher level to you. Although upward comparison can be beneficial when it encourages ambition and inspires people to become more like the people they admire, more often than not it has a negative effect.

How does this relate back to self-esteem? Online, you can take your time to strategically construct a persona that emphasises your most desirable traits and hides any flaws, whereas face-to-face interactions do not allow for the same degree of contemplation or flexibility. On social media, people are far more likely to only share the best aspects of their lives and treat it like a highlight reel. Viewing others' carefully constructed profiles that show a highlight reel of positives appears to diminish our own self-worth. Essentially, when we compare our offline lives with the carefully curated highlights we see online, we fall short. We routinely believe that other people's lives are better than ours, and that people are happier than we are.[103]

This social comparison trap is particularly important in the comparison of bodies. Unsurprisingly, spending more time on social media means more time for body comparisons, which means a higher chance of internalisation of the thin ideal, body dissatisfaction, body shame and disordered eating.[100] Just like in mainstream media, social media sites are a source of images that objectify and oversexualise women, which drives this process further.

Upward comparisons are not just about popularity or appearance; they're also about judging behaviours, such as fitness or eating. There is an idealisation of eating patterns on social media, particularly when linked with moral or personality attributes (e.g. organised, good, healthy). So someone who eats healthily and posts about it on social media by holding a plate of salad next to their abs is likely to be seen as aspirational. There's a reason why 'what I eat in a day' videos have become so popular on YouTube – they're the perfect comparison tool.

Social media provides abundant social comparison opportunities. Before the rise of social media, our social comparison would be limited to school or work hours, and we'd go home and be surrounded by simply our parents (and sometimes siblings). Now we carry our phones in our pockets and have access to social media 24/7, and we use it for an increasing number of tasks and hours in the day. The speed and ease with which we can access information about other people on social media makes for greater opportunity for social comparison. This risks overexposure to upward social comparison information that may have a cumulative detrimental impact on well-being. As a result, it's hardly surprising that more frequent Facebook use has been linked to lower self-esteem in adults, due to increased exposure to upward social comparisons.[104] Also, people who make more social comparisons on social media report greater depressive symptoms, and feel like they are further from their 'ideal self'.

Interestingly, your 'default state' (so to speak) self-esteem level also plays a role, so if you're someone who normally considers themselves to have quite high self-esteem you will generally think of yourself as being more likeable, whereas someone who considers themselves to have low self-esteem will think they are less likeable. Both groups of people, when they feel comfortable and safe, will engage in similar social comparison processes. That is, there's no real difference between them. But add social media into the mix and the differences between these people becomes apparent. When there is a threat to self-image, such as when we are presented with body-ideal images on social media, high-self-esteem individuals are more likely to make a downward social comparison, which raises their self-esteem after the brief dip when they see the images. In contrast, low-self-esteem individuals are more likely to make an upward social comparison, which further lowers their self-esteem.[105] So low mood is amplified, not negated, by going on social media and looking at others, in part due to the social comparison. If you're on your own and looking at social media, then the low-self-esteem individuals definitely have a harder time of it. But in a public group setting – perhaps where you're in a position to compare bodies with peers or you're discussing someone's Instagram account – what this means in practice is that high-self-esteem individuals defend their ego under threat by distancing themselves and becoming more independent, which makes them seem less likeable ('She may have a nicer figure but at least I'm more intelligent.'). The low-self-esteem individuals defend their ego by becoming less independent and more inter-dependent, which makes them more likeable in a group ('Yes, she's more attractive than me, but wow she really does look amazing and happy.'). So even though people with low self-esteem think of themselves as being less likeable, in practice they're actually liked more because of the way they compare and interact with others.

When it comes to Instagram, the audience isn't aware that the content they see may be driven by self-presentation needs (taking pictures of food that you don't eat or enjoy just for the 'likes') and by the creator's own disordered eating behaviour. Following a greater number of strangers on Instagram also leads to greater levels of negative social comparison,[93] which goes a long way to explain the link between Instagram and depression. This social comparison is the key to why social media is linked to issues from depression and anxiety to eating disorders and self-esteem.

The positives

Of course, it's important to note that there are some positives to using social media. The most important of those is communication. These sites allow us to communicate with friends, family, and strangers with similar interests who can become friends. Many people in the Internet generation, including myself, have become real-life friends with people they have met online, and more couples than not now meet through online dating apps. You can meet and engage with people online who are far more diverse than your real-life friendship group, and have discussions with people who think completely differently from you, which can force you to develop your arguments and also see the world from another perspective.

In particular, social media allows people to join a community that they may struggle to find in the real world. Platforms that allow you to post anonymously, such as Tumblr or Instagram, may allow those with social anxiety or other mental health issues to feel less alone. Social media can also be a source of strength and community, for example for LGBTQ+ folks or disabled people who don't see people they can connect with in real life.

Social media also allows people to have a creative outlet and to share that creativity with the world, whether it's art or music. Ideas are developed and shared from creating blogs, podcasts and vlogs. There is even something to be said for the ability to access health information online. People can find out more about subjects such as sexual health and mental health, which they may feel embarrassed to ask about in person or find from a book. Mobile technologies have already produced multiple improvements in healthcare, such as increased medication adherence, better disease understanding and fewer missed appointments.

There is evidence linking social media use with increased

self-esteem, but by a different method not involving social comparison. As mentioned before, when people view their own social media profiles it increases self-esteem, as we are able to view an idealised version of ourselves – our own personal highlight reel.[102] Also, looking at the social media profiles of family and close friends doesn't tend to lower self-esteem, but most of us, especially on Instagram, follow more strangers than friends.

Image-based social media platforms such as Instagram have an additional benefit of decreasing self-reported loneliness to its users, whereas text-based platforms such as Twitter and Facebook don't.[106] Image-based social media platforms may actually mitigate feelings of loneliness because the images give a sense of communicating with an actual person, rather than an object, and allow more insight into a person's life. Humans recognise images much faster than text, which make platforms like Instagram and YouTube seem more personal.

Finally, there's no denying that social media allows for easy sharing of food images and recipes, which can inspire people to try new foods cooked in new ways. Many people now use social media to discover and share food experiences.

Mass mainstream media

Although it is tempting to blame the mass media for perpetuating and glorifying unrealistic standards of physical beauty, the truth is, as always, more complicated than that. Throughout history, the ideal body type has been shaped by society through cultural and political climates, but today we have the addition of the media (including television, film and print), which makes it a far more powerful presence than ever before.

We are surrounded by these media influences daily, so much so that it's impossible for us to be objective and accurate about how much of an influence they have on us. We all like to believe we don't fall for advertising, but if that were the case, companies wouldn't spend huge sums of money on billboards and screen time. They must work.

One incredible study looked at rates of eating disorders in Fiji before and after television was introduced in 1995. Ethnic Fijians have traditionally encouraged healthy appetites and have preferred a rounder, softer body type, as this signified wealth and fertility. Having a strong sense of identity, particularly if tied to culture, can be protective against eating disorders, and this was seen in Fiji as there was only one case of anorexia reported on the island before 1995. But after TV was introduced, rates of dieting shot up from none at all to 69 per cent, people showed clear signs of disordered eating, and they cited attractive actors and actresses on their screens as the inspiration behind their intentions.[107] In follow-up research, it was found that even indirect exposure to mass media increased the risk of disordered eating.[108]

Eating disorders are multifaceted and complex, and it would be a gross oversimplification to suggest that the media is purely responsible for the development of eating disorders, but it's fair to say it plays a role. So why is this?

There are three major core sources of influence that contribute to the development of body image and eating disturbances: parents, peers and the media. These three sources exert their effects through internalisation of societal standards of health and beauty, and through appearance comparison. So the reason the media negatively affects body image is that people will often compare their body with the bodies they are viewing in the media or will internalise the standards of health and beauty that these bodies represent.

Essentially, when you combine a highly lucrative dieting industry with media pressure to look a certain way, increasing rates of eating disorders are obviously concerning, but are also understandable. Cultural standards and ideas of beauty are nothing new, but the impact of the media is a fairly recent addition to this, and is incredibly powerful.

For women, body dissatisfaction results from (and feeds) a system that integrates three fundamental components: idealisation of the thin body, an irrational fear of fat, and a strong belief that weight and shape are key determinants of identity and self-worth. For men, this is becoming a growing problem as well, except with an emphasis on leanness and muscularity over thinness. The media plays a big role in shaping and reinforcing these ideas.

Westernised sociocultural values and focus on the ideal body, which are portrayed through media messages, especially on the Internet, are considered to be a risk factor for the development of disordered eating and eating disorders.[109] Repeated exposure to the depiction of ideal bodies in the media leads to an internalisation of this ideal as normal, realistic and necessary in order to be seen as attractive and desirable. The discrepancy between this ideal and the reality of our own bodily appearance, and how we fall short, leads to body dissatisfaction, low self-esteem and higher risk of eating disorder symptoms. This occurs regardless of the media type.

Interestingly, it seems not all people are affected by the thin ideal in the media, but most are, to the point where it still makes sense for it to be a risk factor.[110] For those who are negatively affected by it, they may be more likely to internalise these ideas and therefore be at risk of disordered eating. Overall, the media influence on women's body image and eating habits appears to be negative.[111]

This makes a lot of sense, and explains why negative body image and disordered eating are consistent phenomena among adults (often young adults) across all ethnicities, social gradients, cultures and countries – the media influence is both influential and omnipresent. It also helps explain why weight and shape concerns and the diet mentality tend to emerge in childhood or young adulthood (as children and teenagers are heavily targeted by the media), why these concerns are so prevalent among young people, and why it's been around for so long that it's considered 'normal' for young people to worry about their weight and body shape.

But if the media is so powerful and omnipresent, and if pretty much all young people are exposed to the content, then why do only a small percentage go on to develop clinical eating disorders? This argument disappears when you consider that the media doesn't act in isolation. Combine this media exposure to the thin ideal with other risk factors – peers talking about weight and body shape, family history of dieting, and reinforcement of the thin ideal by parents or older siblings – and even if we assume that each one has a probability of occurring only in 35 per cent of the population (a very conservative estimate), the probability of all four factors occurring together is 0.35^4, which is 0.015, or 1.5 per cent of the population. Considering it's estimated that 1-2 per cent of the UK population has an eating disorder, it definitely fits.

But while the media certainly has influence over the kinds of bodies we see and are idealised, there is arguably less scope for upward social comparison. Whereas social media is very much peer-based, in newspapers and on television we see more models, celebrities and well-known figures, and these people aren't seen as peers in the same way. There is also greater awareness of the use of editing and airbrushing in traditional media, more so than in social media.

Despite this, there is something about these traditional forms of media that leads us to idolise those who appear and are featured. We see them as being special or noteworthy in some way for being the 'chosen ones' who are accepted to appear on our screens or in the pages we flick through. Especially in today's digital age, there's something exciting about seeing your name or your face in print.

According to studies of adult and adolescent women, exposure to magazines that feature and glamorise the thin ideal is positively correlated with disordered eating.[112] Wanting to look like celebrities and models in the media is a strong predictor of weight concerns, dieting behaviour and binge-eating. A similar study of nearly 800 adolescent girls found that almost 90 per cent said they desired the thin ideal that the media promoted, and as such were more likely to use extreme dieting and disordered eating to try to achieve the ideal.

In television as well, early exposure to the thin ideal leads to an increase in body-image problems years down the line for young girls, regardless of actual or perceived body shape. It affects everyone, no matter their size or ethnicity. The more television a young girl watches, the more likely she is to internalise the thin ideal; and – in adolescence in particular – the more importance a girl places on her appearance, and the more her self-worth is shaped by her body, the more likely she is to have negative body image.

This all comes down to three key facts for girls and young women: first, the perception of pressure from the media to fit the thin ideal is linked to body dissatisfaction. Second, this pressure leads to internalisation of the thin ideal, which means they are more likely to have disordered eating habits. Third, these issues are particularly problematic to the subgroup that are 'high internalisers' – people who are more sensitive to and more affected by the thin ideal, who internalise the ideal more readily by focusing it inwards on themselves, and so are far more likely to feel dissatisfied with their bodies.

Much of the research into the media and body image has focused on women, but there has been a growing interest in the influence on men due to greater awareness of the effect that images of the ideal lean, muscular body can have. Gyms will sell their products and services by displaying pictures of strong, muscular men using their equipment or supplements, and it's highly effective. It persuades men that if they only join that gym or take that supplement, they can look like the man in the image too, even though those particular images, as well as others, are practically unattainable for most people. Over time, these images have become more and more muscular.

Men who feel pressure from traditional media influences to change their body and become more muscular are also more likely to compare their bodies with media images and feel worse about their bodies. These negative feelings mean that these men are more likely to engage in negative behaviours such as increased steroid usage or higher supplement intake, and have an increased chance of developing muscle dysmorphia, bulimia or anorexia nervosa.[113] These behaviours and conditions could lead to health problems or death, including by suicide. Muscle dysmorphia is a growing problem for men in particular; as media images have exerted more pressure, there is a greater chance someone will see their body as 'defective' or 'not big enough'. If the desire to attain this ideal muscular body becomes consuming, then the person may develop great anxiety around their body, which hugely disrupts their life.

In fact, the effect of exposure to the ideal body in the media was similar for men and women – they are all equally affected and made to feel worse about their bodies. It's definitely not just a female thing.

Aside from eating issues and body image, it seems as though excessive media consumption is associated with depression. This definitely seems plausible as there are many different mechanisms by which media exposure could influence the development of depression. For one, spending excessive amounts of time in front of a screen means not being able to spend much time talking to people face-to-face and engage in experiences that are protective against depression, such as exercise. If someone is spending a great deal of time in front of screens at night, then it can displace sleep, which is important for learning and memory, as well as normal emotional development. Another mechanism by which media can more directly lead to depression is by the messages that are internalised from the content viewed. For example, TV shows often present characters and situations that promote ideal body shapes or personality traits, which drive upward social comparison and can lead to low self-esteem. They may also show highly stereotypical portrayals of sociodemographic factors such as sex, ethnicity, sexual orientation and occupation. These stereotypes can interfere with normal identity development and, again, drive social comparison in an unfavourable way. As well as this, what we see on our screens can be very negative or anxiety-provoking, which can lead to a very pessimistic and hopeless view of the world. The combined effect of all of these influences can increase the risk of depression if someone is vulnerable.

Taking all the above together, unsurprisingly the research does show that television exposure and total media exposure are associated with an increased risk of depressive symptoms in young adults, especially in young men.[114] There is also a link between time spent watching TV and use of computer (more than six hours per day) and higher risk of depression in adults.[115] Television in particular tends to feature a large amount of advertising, where the purpose is to make the viewer feel their life is inadequate unless they purchase the items on the screen.

On the flipside, people do use media such as video games and watch TV as a social activity, which can negate some of the negatives. There are also certain types of television content that can actually reduce the risk of depression. Humour, which is an integral part of many shows, tends to result in laughter, and laughter can reduce stress and lift mood. This doesn't seem to apply when someone is already in the depths of depression, though. Individuals with depression may spend more time watching TV due to the social isolation and lack of energy, irrespective of whether their viewing habits contributed to the onset of their depression.

Aside from mental health, spending too much time watching television has an impact on our physical health, because if you're spending several hours per day watching TV you're also likely sitting down for that whole time. This sedentary behaviour, i.e. sitting down for hours on end, is related to higher risk of heart disease and death, regardless of how much physical activity you do. This is partly because being too sedentary can increase signs of inflammation and stress in your body.[116] I don't say this in order to scare you out of watching any TV at all, just to highlight that, as always, too much of anything isn't ideal – especially if your job requires you to sit down for most of the day.

The positives

It's easy to see the media as a highly negative influence on our health, especially our mental health. But there are some positives to note.

Exposure to media outlets can help you to understand the world around you, how different people live, and in general what's happening outside your immediate environment. For children, television shows can be educational and provide teaching moments. A great example of this is *Sesame Street*, where young children can learn about simple arithmetic, the alphabet, kindness, and even complicated issues such as disability and race.

Video games get a lot of bad press, but there's some good in them too, particularly as some can help people develop and fine-tune their motor skills and coordination.

It's important to note that the Internet, with everything that comes with it, including media and social media, provides something that is accessible to people with disabilities, allows people with mental health issues to access help from the comfort of their homes, and is a safer route for people seeking aid from domestic abuse than a phone, as it's easier to erase proof.

Overall, there are some positives to the media, but, as you might have already noticed, this section is quite short compared with the potential negative impacts.

Overall, exposure to thin- and lean-ideal media has many negative effects: it's linked with greater body dissatisfaction and self-criticism, lower self-esteem, negative mood, disordered eating, more self-consciousness, higher weight-related appearance anxiety, and feelings of depression, shame and guilt. That's pretty damning.

Misinformation and the rise of Netflix

The biggest issue with media and social media is the widespread availability of misinformation: 42 per cent of American adult social media users have said that the information they find on social media would affect health decisions related to diet, exercise or stress management, and nearly 90 per cent of people aged eighteen to twenty-four years have indicated they would trust medical information found on social media. To me, that is more than slightly worrying.

There is no real regulation of the information and advice given on the Internet, where anyone can portray themselves as an expert and conflicts of interest are hidden away. Social media undoubtedly plays a key role in this, and this is now being discussed extensively. But what hasn't been talked about enough is the role of documentaries with blatant agendas, and the role of streaming services such as Netflix in circulating these to a huge audience.

What the Health, Fat, Sick and Nearly Dead, The Magic Pill, GMO OMG... There is an ever-increasing number available online.

Documentaries such as *What the Health* don't really deserve to be called documentaries. They are propaganda pieces that twist available evidence, cite 'expert' opinions and use emotive fearmongering language to further their respective agendas, all under the guise of informing with impartiality. These programmes are so relentlessly terrifying that by the end you want to immediately change your entire way of eating, convinced that particular foods will certainly kill you and cause you great harm. They aren't documentaries so much as horror movies.

What the Health has a highly specific agenda: it promotes the vegan diet as the answer to preventing and curing pretty much all disease; any foods that don't fit this mould (eggs, dairy, meat, fish) are viciously portrayed as the enemy, and this information they've 'uncovered' (ha) is all being hidden by Big Food*, who are trying to keep you from the truth.

It's also highly hypocritical: conflicts of interest that serve the agenda are highlighted, but they don't acknowledge that pretty much everyone they interview also has conflicts of interest, whether it's their diet books or supplements or activism work. While this isn't enough, I would argue, to completely discredit

---

*   You know, those large industrial food producers and manufacturers who only care about profits and apparently have unwavering unlimited power over our food supply? Those guys.

what they say, bias is still bias, and it should go both ways. But instead of being impartial, these documentaries can't instil a single ounce of doubt, and so instead go for a massive double standard that further reduces their credibility.

Contrast this with *The Magic Pill*, which promotes a ketogenic/paleo diet that is very low in total carbohydrates, high in fat and high in animal products. This is a diet that is arguably the polar opposite of veganism, yet if you were to watch both programmes (and I highly recommend you don't), you'd see some surprising similarities between the two.

First, both have a very simple solution to the complex issue that is what we should eat. Go vegan! Avoid sugar! Eat fat! Only juice! There is only one right way to eat for health and any evidence to support any other way must be totally ignored. Second, they both rely on celebrities and doctors (or nutritional therapists) who vehemently support this one way of eating and who will say only positive, supportive things about it, even if they're wrong. These are the kind of doctors who usually don't see patients one-to-one, who sell diet books and/or supplements online, and who are deeeeeefinitely not biased in any way. Anecdotes and testimonials are far more powerful at persuading the public than endless studies, so getting some of those in certainly helps. Third, they use the most outrageous language to induce fear. Toxins! Chemicals! Epidemic! Disaster! Deadly! It's important to make the situation sound as dire as possible. This is then accompanied by the usual stigmatising images of fat people walking, eating the scary food, and fat building up in the body.

Most food documentaries are bad because nutrition science isn't definitive. But we like the simple narrative of 'X food causes

Y disease', even though it's incredibly difficult to determine causality in nutrition research. These documentaries take complex messages of potential associations and simplify them to suggest that there are good foods that prevent disease and bad foods that cause disease, and this is all you need to know.

Yes, the dramatic and emotional effect of the stories does have an impact and a purpose, and it succeeds. Their main goal is for you to change and to feel bad about not changing. One of the dangers of these kinds of documentaries is that they scare people into making drastic food decisions, which they then either abandon just as quickly for another fad, or which they maintain out of fear, where any transgression causes immense anxiety, leaving them in a situation very much reminiscent of orthorexia. Drastic dietary changes like that, unless supervised by a medical professional, are risky as they are poorly researched, which means a higher likelihood of deficiencies and ill effects. For example, one of the 'experts' in *What the Health* states that you can get all your protein requirements from eating 2,000 calories worth of rice, which completely ignores the fact that rice doesn't contain amino acids in the right proportions, and this would (over time) result in a lack of leucine in the diet. And anyone stupid enough to compare eggs to smoking shouldn't be allowed to give medical advice. *The Magic Pill* even goes so far as to suggest a ketogenic diet can cure cancer – an incredibly dangerous suggestion.

Almost all these documentaries are set in the US and focus on the US food supply, which is quite different from the UK, from Europe and from Australia. Everything they say about the food supply and about food manufacturing should be taken with a pinch of salt, and you definitely shouldn't assume it's the same here.

Netflix health documentaries don't help us be healthier or help our understanding about health. They confuse what we know about nutrition science and obscure the truths of nutrition that could actually help us live healthier lives.

Conclusion

Whether you are impacted by the media and social media in a positive or negative way, or barely at all, depends on a complex interplay between individual personal characteristics and the larger social climate. Most of the time, negative media effects are not intended, of course. Most media producers and social media influencers aren't trying to harm people, but that doesn't absolve them from responsibility when the content they produce has negative effects.

Also, don't get your nutrition information from sensationalist documentary film-makers.

Quiz: Do you have social media anxiety disorder?

Check how many of these common symptoms of social media anxiety disorder you identify with:

	YES/NO
Interrupting conversations to check your social media accounts	
Lying to others about how much time you spend on social media	
Withdrawal from friends and family	
Trying to stop or reduce your use of social media more than once before without being successful	
Loss of interest in other activities	
Neglecting work or school to comment on Facebook or Twitter account	
Experiencing withdrawal symptoms when you are not able to access social media	
Spending over six hours per day on social networking sites like Facebook, Twitter or Instagram	
Overwhelming need to share things with others on social media sites	
Having your phone with you 24 hours a day to check your social media sites	
Using social media more often than you planned	
Severe nervousness or anxiety when you are not able to check your notifications	
Negative impacts on your personal or professional life due to social media usage	

The more of these you identify with, the more likely it is that you may have some anxieties around social media and should perhaps look into reducing your usage.

Quiz: How does the media affect your body image?

Please read each of the following points carefully and indicate the number that best reflects your agreement with the statement.

	DEFINITELY DISAGREE	MOSTLY DISAGREE	NEITHER AGREE NOR DISAGREE	MOSTLY AGREE	DEFINITELY AGREE
I've felt pressure from TV or magazines to lose weight.	1	2	3	4	5
I compare my body with the bodies of people who are on TV.	1	2	3	4	5
I would like my body to look like the models who appear in magazines.	1	2	3	4	5
I would like my body to look like the people who are in films.	1	2	3	4	5
I've felt pressure from TV or magazines to have a perfect body.	1	2	3	4	5
I've felt pressure from TV or magazines to exercise.	1	2	3	4	5
I compare my body with that of people who are athletic.	1	2	3	4	5
I've felt pressure from TV or magazines to change my appearance.	1	2	3	4	5

The higher your score, the more you rely on the media and societal ideals to shape your ideas about your body and weight.

8

EXERCISE, FITSPO AND BODY IMAGE

*'Beauty is about being comfortable in your own skin.
It's about knowing and accepting who you are.'*

ELLEN DEGENERES

I remember the first time I walked into one of these popular fitness and wellness festivals in London. Immediately I was surrounded by people dressed in Lycra, giant posters advertising every protein supplement under the sun, and the sounds of an instructor shouting at a group to 'Push harder! Feel the burn! If you're not sweating you might as well not be here!' The instant feeling of inadequacy was intense.

Exercise is, undoubtedly, one of the key aspects of health. But the fitness industry is primarily focused on aesthetics. Just look at the most popular fitness accounts on Instagram. They're not necessarily the fittest or healthiest – they're the people with the most aesthetically pleasing bodies. They're attractive people with flat stomachs (preferably visible abs), small waists and perfectly round behinds.

Alongside the changing trends in what we should and shouldn't be eating, there has been a confusing, ever-changing landscape of popularity in fitness. Boutique indoor cycling studios compete with outdoor boot-camp classes, yoga, Pilates, barre, CrossFit, and all manner of high-intensity interval training (HIIT) classes. These HIIT classes all compete to be the hardest workout in existence – the workout that burns the most calories, or the class that'll get you shredded the fastest. It's extreme, it's aggressive and it's intimidating.

Fitspo

If you've spent some time on social media recently, you'll see the trend for 'strong, not skinny'.

The rise of 'fitspiration' or 'fitspo' has primarily been on Instagram. These are images of aspirational fitness (fitness + inspiration = fitspiration), and as they are images, they are heavily focused on aesthetics. There are millions and millions of fitspo images on Instagram. The term is a play on the term 'thinspiration', which is often found on pro-anorexia sites. But where thinspiration websites support and encourage weight loss and eating disorders, fitspiration supposedly advocates a fit and healthy lifestyle. The question, though, is whether fitspo is really just a more socially acceptable form of thinspo. Fitspo aligns itself perfectly with societal ideals of health – for women it's seeking the thin ideal, while for men it's the lean, muscular ideal. And it plays perfectly into societal ideals of youth and beauty, reinforcing these ideas to vulnerable people. You would expect that a highly unattainable fit ideal would have a similarly negative effect to the extreme and equally unattainable thin ideal of thinspo. And it does: both types of content end up being surprisingly similar, with themes of dieting and restriction, weight stigma and guilt-inducing messages.[117]

Fitspo is designed to motivate someone to exercise and to feel good about themselves, but it achieves the exact opposite. The majority of fitspo images feature just one body type: thin and toned,[118] which adds to the narrative that fitness can only look one way, and if you look different, then fitness isn't for you. In trying to be inspirational, fitspo ends up excluding people, worsening people's body image and contributing to lower self-esteem, so people feel worse about themselves for not matching up to this ideal fitness standard.[119] In addition, fitspiration sexually objectifies the fit body, with text and images encouraging people to see themselves as objects or ornaments, and ignoring bodily signals like pain. Despite apparently being focused on fitness, the actual focus of fitspo is more on the body as an object to be admired than a body that can move.

How many posters or Instagram captions have you seen that show this, whether it's the controversial Protein World ad that asked 'Are you beach body ready?', or a fitness studio telling you pain is weakness leaving the body, or a fitness blogger posting a photo where they've distorted and twisted their body into the most aesthetically and sexually appealing position – usually emphasising the tiny waist relative to the 'booty gains'. Half of fitspo images of women don't even include their face: the whole focus is on the body.

Although fitspo and the 'strong, not skinny' movement had good intentions, it still very much sits neatly within the societal beauty ideal and being completely in control of your health and weight. The desire for a seriously fit-looking body is just a variation on the desire for a thin body. It may be disguised as being health-focused, but it's ill-advised as it still values a single body type as being better and being worth more, and it's especially problematic when that body type is impossible for most people to achieve. In the end, it's arguably just another way to shame men and women who don't fit into this unrealistic ideal.

For the followers of fitspo this is additionally problematic, as by following or liking these pictures we're publicly endorsing this fit ideal body shape, making it personal. This makes it gain further importance in our minds, as it then goes beyond simply representing a societal ideal; it also represents our personal ideal. Then every time we fall short of this ideal, when we compare ourselves with these images or people, it becomes a personal failure. And that hurts more. It exacerbates the negative effects on our self-worth. On top of that, the popularity of these images then just strengthens the narrative that this is the ideal body through endorsement from others – we can see which images on Instagram have the most likes or the most comments. And this reinforces the idea that this *should* be our personal goal.

Unlike the images we tend to see on television or on magazine covers, these images of the fit ideal aren't just celebrities and models – they're people just like us, with jobs and commitments, who haven't been Photoshopped or airbrushed (we assume). As we discussed in the chapter on social media, this makes us feel that these are peers who are good people to compare ourselves with, and that upward social comparison doesn't end well.

Once someone who posts fitspo sees that their body is giving them external validation in the form of likes and follows, it's hard to resist. So much so that the people posting this kind of content are more likely to have disordered eating behaviour and unhealthy, obsessive attitudes towards exercise.[120] While giving the illusion of absolute health and well-being, it turns out these people are not necessarily healthy at all. In pursuit of achieving and maintaining the 'ideal' fit body shape, they've sacrificed their mental health.

Most important, perhaps, is the fact that these posts and images, despite their intentions to motivate, do not lead people to exercise more.[121] In fact, it may lead people to exercise less due to the negative effects on body image and self-esteem.[122]

Benefits of exercise

The benefits of exercise go far beyond simply aesthetics. To reduce exercise and movement down to simply appearance does it a huge disservice. The link between exercise and focus on aesthetics often boils down to exercise being used as a tool for weight loss, while other health benefits are just ignored or not seen as important enough. In almost any research on exercise, body weight is used as the measure of success or failure, and most people who sign up for the gym or personal training cite this as their goal. If weight loss doesn't happen, it's not that the exercise didn't work (because everybody knows of course it works), it's that the person didn't do everything they were supposed to, they didn't try hard enough, or they overcompensated by eating more. In other words, the blame is placed on the individual for failing to lose weight.

Experiencing higher levels of hunger after exercise is a normal biological response that happens to most people. This is why exercise isn't a magic bullet for weight loss, despite what we've been told. When you exercise, your body demands more energy; it increases your hunger signals, and so you eat more. That's not a personal failure, that's responding to basic bodily signals. And as we've already seen, fighting hunger signals and fighting biology just doesn't work.

If someone embarks on an exercise programme that doesn't lead to significant (or any) weight loss, they're more likely to give up because they believe that it hasn't worked, it hasn't helped. This is totally the wrong way to look at exercise, and I by no means wish to blame people who have experienced this. I think it's totally understandable, it's the fault of how we as a society have fixated on weight above every other measure of health. Having a wider, more transparent view of the benefits of exercise is so important. The effectiveness of exercise shouldn't be judged exclusively on changes in body weight. There are so many other incredible physiological and psychological benefits to exercise, independent of weight loss.

Regular exercise lowers general risk of dying prematurely and can prevent the onset of type 2 diabetes, high blood pressure and heart disease. Regular exercise has a considerable positive effect on markers of health and various risk factors for disease, such as reduced blood triglyceride levels, more favourable cholesterol levels and reduced blood pressure,[123] all of which decreases the chance of developing heart disease. There is also a positive effect on blood sugar balance, which reduces the chance of developing type 2 diabetes, independently of weight loss.[124]

The type of exercise can also play a role. For example, aerobic exercise such as running can reduce resting heart rate and blood pressure, as well as improve mood.[125]

In older adults, particularly women after menopause, bone mineral density gradually decreases. This is an inevitable part of ageing and means that postmenopausal women are more likely to get fractures and broken bones. Long term, exercise is associated with decreased fracture incidence and slower decrease in bone mineral density in elderly women.[126] You can't stop the loss of bone mineral density, but exercise can at least slow it down.

Cognitive decline is another unfortunate aspect of ageing. Research on the effects of exercise on cognition and Alzheimer's disease – the most common type of dementia – show that movement is highly beneficial. For example, in one study, 1,740 people over the age of 65 were asked about the number of times per week they had exercised for at least 15 minutes over the last year. After 6 years, there were far more patients with Alzheimer's in the group who didn't do any exercise, compared with those who exercised at least three times per week. Other studies have reported similar positive effects of exercise on dementia.[127]

There are several proposed biological explanations for this, including increased blood flow to the brain and dopamine release. But these don't really explain why there are differences between groups of people – for example, why exercise has a stronger positive effect on women than men, and why the positive effects of exercise seem to increase with age, so someone aged 70 would get more benefit than someone age 60. For now, we don't know the full explanation as to why exercise helps, but we can be sure that it does.

It's important to note that these kinds of health markers (cholesterol levels, blood pressure, bone density, etc.) are not obviously accessible to most people, whereas weight is far more obvious and easier to measure. Sadly, this means that most people are effectively blind to these benefits, and won't realise when they occur. Not losing weight does not mean that exercise hasn't had any benefit.

With all these incredible benefits to our physical health, it's no wonder that being active and moving our bodies means we're less likely to die sooner and more likely to live longer, healthier lives. But what about mental health?

Mental health

You'll often see memes on Facebook that claim you shouldn't take pills for depression – you should go for a run instead! Or a slightly different one with an image of nature saying, 'This is an antidepressant,' followed by an image of a pill with the text 'This is shit.' Not only is this pill-shaming, which is incredibly unhelpful and stigmatising, but it's also a massive over-statement of the evidence.

There does seem to be a link between exercise and mental health, and it's worth exploring, as many people report that running in particular helps clear their head and provides a distraction from the anxieties and stresses of everyday life.

Doing some form of exercise is consistently linked to better mental health outcomes. People who engage in regular exercise are less likely to experience depression and anxiety years down the line. There is also growing evidence that exercise can help reduce the symptoms of depression.[128] These effects seem to be greatest in those with treatment-resistant depression, and it can take up to eight to twelve weeks to really see significant changes in symptoms. While the exact duration and amount of exercise needed will depend on the person, it seems that as little as one hour per week can produce benefits,[129] and it doesn't even seem to matter what type of exercise is done, whether it's aerobic (running) or nonaerobic (strength training or yoga). What matters is that it has to be consistent and fairly regular.

But we should be hesitant about suggesting that lack of exercise causes depression, or that exercise can treat depression. Depression is complex and often related to issues such as trauma, low self-esteem and stress, which exercise doesn't get to the root of. Movement can be extremely beneficial for distracting the mind, but it can't necessarily process traumatic events in the same way that therapy can. It's also important to note that some individuals, for medical reasons or due to disability, are unable or not advised to exercise. In cases of severe depression in particular, someone might need medication to even get to the point where they feel they can exercise, otherwise they may be in such a low place that any kind of activity feels like too much. The benefits of exercise in depression are real and significant, but don't negate the importance of appropriate treatment using medication or talking therapy.

One possible partial explanation for the link between nature/running and depression is vitamin D. Research shows that there is a link between symptoms of depression and low levels of vitamin D in the body.[130] However, what the research doesn't show is whether low vitamin D levels cause depression, whether low vitamin D levels occur because of depression, or whether there's some other explanation involved. It's possible that low vitamin D levels is one of many factors that contribute to someone feeling depressed, but it's also possible that people who have depression go outdoors less, and so have low vitamin D levels because of that. (A quick reminder: our bodies make vitamin D in response to activation by UV rays from the sun, which cannot penetrate glass.) It has been suggested that a vitamin D supplement could be beneficial for someone with depression, but only if they were deficient to begin with. It wouldn't help someone who already has vitamin D levels within the normal range.

There has been quite a lot of interest in the link between exercise and depression, but less so with anxiety disorders. That exercise can help with depression has pretty much reached the level of 'it's common sense', likely because it's been spoken about more, and also because the clinical diversity of anxiety disorders doesn't allow for generalisation across the board. What works for social anxiety won't be the same as for post-traumatic stress disorder (PTSD) or panic disorder.

There is some evidence to suggest that exercise and move-ment can help with some forms of anxiety and panic disorder,[128] but just as with depression, it is not a cure. If people are on a waiting list to receive talking therapy for anxiety, doing some form of movement, particularly running, can be something to help in the meantime.

Although we've reached a point where it seems obvious that exercising does benefit mental health, we're still not entirely sure why there are benefits. It's likely to be a complex interaction of psychological and neurobiological mechanisms that work together to mediate the link between exercise and depression or anxiety disorders. The majority of the protective effects of exercise against depression occur within the first hour of exercise undertaken each week, which provides some clues. Some suggestions have been put forward, such as increased social support, a sense of mastery, independence, achievement and distraction. These are mainly psychological, and in addition there are suggested biological pathways such as the role of serotonin, changes in the hypothalamic adrenocortical system, which is involved in the stress response, and endorphins.

When you exercise, your body releases chemicals called endorphins, which interact with receptors in your brain that reduce your perception of pain. Endorphins also trigger a positive feeling in the body, similar to that of morphine. Endorphins get their name from morphine, as they are endogenous morphine-like substances (endo – orphins) that produce pain relief. After around twenty to thirty minutes of moderately hard exercise, endorphins are released into your body and will result in a mood and energy boost for two to three hours, and a mild buzz for up to twenty-four hours. This is what's generally known as 'runner's high'.

Other explanations for any association between exercise and depression and anxiety focus on the fact that exercise results in improved physical health, as well as affecting self-esteem.

Self-esteem and exercise is an interesting kettle of fish. While it may seem like there should be a really obvious link – namely that exercise increases self-esteem – that doesn't seem to be the case. The research is really mixed, with around 60 per cent of studies showing a positive link,[131] suggesting that exercise does help for some groups of people, whereas for others it makes no difference. The lack of a general trend indicates that there is no one simple explanation for the link between exercise and self-esteem, but rather that there are several. For example, for those with disabilities the effects of exercise are often overwhelmingly positive, likely due to the autonomy and personal control this gives. There may also be that sense of belonging to a group, which can help relieve loneliness and improve self-esteem. Exercise also seems to be incredibly beneficial for those in larger bodies, as often the stigma and microaggressions associated with this mean that self-esteem is very low to begin with, so there is more scope for subtle but significant improvement. Also, those who are sedentary are more likely to experience positive changes in self-esteem, as they are more likely to see changes in physical fitness, which can make it seem like the exercise is 'working', i.e. leading to body changes.

Even for those without depression or anxiety, there are considerable benefits of exercise for stress management. Just around twenty minutes of movement per day is enough to have stress-relieving effects, and that includes things like walking or gardening.[132] For me, for example, that's equivalent to walking to the nearest train station and back again.

Factors that I've already mentioned, like endorphins and the social aspect of exercise, definitely seem to contribute to this. In addition, stress can result in holding tension in particular areas of the body such as the shoulders, and exercise can help with this by forcing those muscles to tense and relax. Many forms of exercise also require a level of concentration, whether that's focusing on breathing in yoga, or playing a game of tennis, which distracts the mind away from sources of stress and frustration.

Something about being in nature is especially calming for us humans. Brain scans have shown that simply looking at photos of natural scenes can have a calming effect. Walking outside in nature (as opposed to along a busy road) lowers levels of cortisol – the stress hormone – and seems to encourage us to slow down our breathing rate. Out of the people who say stress management is their primary motivation for exercise, most prefer running, walking or yoga, and two out of three of those usually take place outdoors.

Interestingly, people's motivations for movement seem to differ based on the type. Motivation for playing a sport seems to be more inward, such as enjoyment and a challenge, whereas the motivation for engaging in exercise is more outward, with a focus on weight loss and appearance.[133]

This is worrying for two main reasons. First, we have already established that weight loss is an unattainable and unrealistic goal for the vast majority. When it comes to exercise in particular, the increased movement and energy expenditure usually results in a biological drive to increase hunger and therefore eat more, which would negate any kind of calorie deficit that would lead to weight loss. This isn't 'lack of willpower', this is fighting biology, and so understandably it's fighting a losing battle. So, when embarking on an exercise regime doesn't lead to weight loss (due to biology), people are likely to become disheartened and give up, despite the fact that exercise has a whole host of amazing benefits beyond weight loss, which I've just spent several pages outlining. They miss out on all these amazing benefits, simply because society tells us that weight matters above all else.

Second, focusing on appearance and aesthetics, and in particular focusing on obtaining the thin or lean ideal, has led to an increase in body-image disturbance in individuals across the gender spectrum. Negative body image is a key part of (and a predictor of) a variety of health issues such as depression, eating disorders and body dysmorphic disorder (BDD).

The most popular theory, and the one with the most support and evidence, which explains how body-image disturbance comes to be and how it's maintained, is sociocultural theory. This theory states that social pressures (such as from the media, friends and family) are a trigger for people to conform to the thin or lean ideal. For the vast majority of people, this ideal is difficult or even impossible to achieve, even with regular exercise, so it's not surprising that improving body image and obtaining this ideal is a strong motivator for doing some form of exercise.

People who do some kind of exercise generally have better body image than people who don't. But why? This is where it gets really interesting. Those who exercise seem to be more likely to be close to societal ideals of body shape, and therefore may have more external influences that validate their body. For men, doing mainly weight training has the most effect, whereas for women it's a mixture of cardio and weights. Both of these lead to the same goal: reaching the ideal. Doing weights builds the muscle for the lean, muscular ideal for men; and doing cardio and weights allows women to reach the thin ideal (not too many muscles, God forbid). It may also be because exercise is associated with a whole host of psychological benefits. We can't be sure, and it likely differs from person to person. But what we do know is that exercising directly causes better body image for many people, which is amazing.[134] This effect doesn't apply as much to older adults, though, particularly over age fifty-five, which is likely down to loss of function and reduced ability to move in the same way as when they were younger, rather than due to appearance, although it's possible that society's definition of beauty being young and wrinkle-free may be contributing as well. Of course, this is totally understandable. If you feel like your body isn't working as well as you want it to, and at the same time you're bombarded with images of youthful beauty, how would that not make you feel worse about your own body?

It's clear that there are mental health benefits associated with exercise, but that's definitely not always the case. As always, it's a little more nuanced than that. For some people, exercise ends up making them feel worse, and this is down to the ideas and perceptions we have about exercise.

The reason that someone exercises or moves their body is what dictates the relationship between body and self-esteem and disordered eating. In particular, exercising in order to lose weight or to appear more attractive (by being closer to the thin ideal) is why some women become more dissatisfied with their body when they exercise, regardless of any physical and psychological benefits. This is likely because exercise doesn't change your body overnight; it takes time, it's slow, it's painful and it's challenging. It's demotivating when this hard work doesn't produce a quick reward and doesn't quickly bring someone closer to the thin ideal, as we're led to believe it's us and our body that's the problem. When the motivation is weight and aesthetics, the result is worse body image, whereas when the motivation is health, particularly mental health, the result is better body image.

One interesting way in which we can understand this relationship between body image and motivation to exercise is 'objectification theory'. This theory is based on the idea that within our culture women are constantly looked at, assessed and objectified. What is deemed to be feminine and attractive is what gains the approval of the male gaze – a focus on the body as an object to be admired. This regular objectification can lead to a process called self-objectification, whereby women internalise these ideas and outsiders' perspectives, which results in placing high value on aesthetics and appearance. Naturally, this needs constant monitoring and produces high anxiety about the body, which is why it leads to body dissatisfaction, body shame, lower self-esteem, disordered eating and depression.

For many people, when they embark on an exercise programme or they want to spend an hour moving their body, they'll go to a gym or studio of some sort. This kind of fitness environment provides an ideal atmosphere for self-objectification, as there are mirrors all around, there are posters showing thin women doing exercises, 'before' and 'after' pictures emphasising weight loss, classes with names like 'ultimate fat burn', and plenty of other women's bodies in tight-fitting Lycra to compare themselves with. All highly objectifying.

There is such a clear divide between the messages in gyms directed at men compared with women. For women, weight-loss programmes are advertised by focusing on slimness and thinness, using words such as 'Slimacise', whereas for men it's much more aggressive: 'Axe Fat', or 'Project Hench' for those looking to build muscle. For women, there is no focus on muscle gain; instead it's all about 'shaping' and 'toning' the body, moulding it as if it were an inanimate object that needs fixing.

Within that kind of environment there are several difference types of fitness activity to choose from. There are individual workouts where you can choose cardio or weights, and there are group fitness classes such as aerobics, weights-based classes and yoga. Different workouts seem to have different effects on body image. In general, cardio workouts place an emphasis on burning fat and burning calories, and so tend to be quite weight-loss-focused, rather than emphasising the benefits of improved cardiovascular fitness. So, many women who do cardio-based exercises or classes do so to lose weight, which usually leads to greater body dissatisfaction, because the focus is purely on aesthetics. Weights-based workouts, on the other hand, don't have that same emphasis, but instead focus on functional strength and fitness, which doesn't lead to greater body image concerns. Yoga-based exercise has a different focus again, emphasising the mind–body connection, increasing body awareness, and breath work. The lack of emphasis on aesthetics is protective against self-objectification and leads to better body image.[135]

It is interesting to note that participating in cardio-based group fitness classes is associated with exercising more for enjoyment and mood improvement, whereas this isn't the case for individual cardio workouts. Group classes have a reputation for being more enjoyable and social occasions, and research has shown that in general women prefer to exercise in group settings rather than alone (although of course everyone is different). Combine that with the upbeat music and motivational instructors and it's no wonder many people see these classes as being more fun.

What this practically means is that gyms and fitness studios need to focus on functional reasons for exercise, such as health, fitness, enjoyment and better mood, rather than focusing on appearance-related reasons such as weight loss. That would go a long way towards improving women's body image. But of course they won't do that. Focusing on aesthetics and weight loss is what brings in lots of new customers and members, and fitness studios thrive on unrealistic societal beauty standards, as it keeps people coming back. What may be a more realistic goal is suggesting that gyms create a more positive environment in gyms, by reducing the number of mirrors, removing objectifying and unrealistic posters of women's bodies, employing staff with diverse body shapes and sizes, and instructing staff to focus on promoting benefits and motivations for exercise that aren't appearance-focused. Anything but shouting about how many calories someone is burning during a class.

Body dissatisfaction isn't something that's unique to women, as has been thought in the past. Men are just as likely to be dissatisfied with their bodies, but in a different way. Most women are keen to reduce their body weight, whereas men are split pretty evenly down the middle, with half wanting to lose weight and half wanting to gain weight, but always with the intention of achieving the ideal body shape.[136] This body dissatisfaction is linked with pursuing exercise for aesthetic goals, which only seems to further negative body image, as the ideal body shape is unattainable for most people.

Ideally, we need to totally shift the argument about exercise away from aesthetics, to improve body image. Another reason this is important is the risk of overexercise.

Overexercise

In the 1970s the concept of 'positive addiction' was introduced, using exercise as an example. It was thought that whereas with substance abuse and other addictions there was a negative relationship whereby taking more would consistently decrease health, with exercise it seemed that the more you took, the better your health. I'm sure you can already see the problem with this, and these ideas were soon challenged by other psychologists, who had seen patients who exercised to the point of persistent physical injury and to the detriment of their family and social lives. They were spending so much time exercising they had no energy for their families.

Just as with other forms of addiction, excessive exercise behaviour becomes problematic when someone experiences withdrawal symptoms if they are unable to exercise for more than a day or two, experiences feelings of guilt and anxiety if a workout is missed combined with reduced anxiety immediately after a workout, and when the level of exercise interferes with other activities, such as sleep or social life, in a detrimental way. This can also include exercising despite medical advice not to, for example due to injury.[137] This hopefully clears up any confusion between commitment to exercise and actual overexercise or exercise addiction. Someone who is simply committed to improving their mental health or running a marathon for charity shouldn't be experiencing high levels of anxiety and letting it take over their lives. It should simply mesh in with other aspects of life, and become part of a routine, rather than overwhelming.

Personally, I prefer the term 'overexercise' as it's less scary and stigmatising than the word 'addiction', and that way I can also include those who exercise too much but who would still be considered subclinical. Using the word 'addiction' can feel like over-medicalising the problem and put people off potentially changing their behaviour to something more moderate and positive, as they don't see themselves as being addicted.

Overexercise can be a problem unique in itself, or it can be a secondary outcome of another issue, such as an eating disorder. The former – primary exercise addiction – typically involves avoiding a negative outcome such as stress or anxiety, whereas the latter generally involves using exercise as a means to lose weight. The main difference between the two is that in primary exercise addiction, the exercise is the objective, whereas in secondary exercise addiction, weight loss is the objective, with overexercise being one of the key ways to achieve that goal.

The two may have different causes, but the symptoms presented are usually the same, or very similar. Most of the time, overexercising comes together with some form of disordered eating behaviour.

In the UK, it has been suggested that around 3 per cent of people are at risk of overexercise.[138] This may not sound like much, but actually adds up to a significant number of people. To put that into context, anorexia nervosa is suggested to affect around 1 per cent of the population.

There are several explanations as to why overexercise develops, but in reality it's likely an overlap of many factors. First, there is the endorphin hypothesis, which suggests that 'runner's high' and that feeling of euphoria can encourage addictive behaviour. Second, there is the suggestion that because your body temperature increases when you exercise it helps you relax, and this reduces anxiety in an ever more addicting way. A less purely biological explanation is that exercise becomes a mechanism to cope with stress to the point where someone can become dependent on it as their only stress reliever.

Someone who is exercising in a healthy way is generally motivated by positive reinforcement – the reward of exercise, whether it's physical, mental or social, is what they are seeking. Someone overexercising in an unhealthy way has this too, but with an additional component of negative reinforcement –

they're trying to avoid the unpleasant feelings of guilt and anxiety that make up the withdrawal symptoms of missing a workout or two. So rather than simply wanting to exercise, there's a feeling of 'I *have* to exercise.'

For some people, that negative reinforcement is driven by body dysmorphic disorder (BDD), which could be either quite mild or very severe. Individuals with BDD have a distorted body image and a preoccupation with perceived defects with the body, and any existing imperfections are seen as being far greater than they actually are. These imperfections can be things like scars, blemishes or a lack of symmetry – things that someone else might not even notice. BDD can present itself in the form of a variety of negative behaviours, from time-consuming rituals such as constantly checking appearance in the mirror, to social isolation, overexercise and higher risk of depression. Muscle dysmorphia is a version of BDD that specifically focuses on a perception that a person isn't muscular enough, that they're too small. It is this group that is most likely to overexercise – particularly excessive weight-lifting, which can damage joints and muscles – as well as abuse diuretics and steroids to achieve a more muscular look.[139] Muscle dysmorphia is absolutely driven by societal body ideals, as the more someone internalises this ideal, the more likely they are to pursue muscularity as an important goal.[140] But there is also a worry about how other people perceive your body, and whether it's seen as good enough, which is known as social physique anxiety.

The difficulty with overexercise or exercise addiction is that many people don't see it as a problem. It is likely that exercise is viewed by society as being kind of a necessity for healthy living, and as such it is viewed positively by both society and individuals. Exercising many hours a day is seen as being more 'normal' and socially acceptable than spending many hours a day playing video games, especially in the eyes of parents.

Of course, everyone who exercises is on a spectrum, ranging from a healthy relationship with exercise to a full exercise addiction, and where you draw the cut-off line between clinical and 'normal' is tricky, especially as fitness and exercising is seen as a positive thing, and is encouraged by family and friends, even when it is obsessive and unhealthy.

Yes, exercise is highly beneficial to both mental and physical health, but it's not simply a case of 'the more the better'. Exercise and movement shouldn't take over your life, nor should people be made to feel guilty if there are factors preventing them from exercising, such as disability or finance. The amazing benefits of exercise should be presented to us with a warning that losing control and overdoing it can potentially be as dangerous as misusing any other behaviour or substance. The body needs to recover after exercise through carefully planned rest periods, which are just as important as the workout itself. As always, moderation is key.

The positives of fitspo

I think it's important to acknowledge that fitspo isn't all bad. For some people, having a visual diary to post their fitness content keeps them motivated to pursue their goals in a healthy way. For others, viewing fitspo content genuinely does motivate them in a positive way, rather than due to negative social comparisons and feeling not good enough.

Young girls in particular have a complicated relationship with exercise. Girls generally are less active than boys, and the amount of activity they do as they get older declines faster than for boys. Part of this is down to the fact that for girls, especially adolescent girls, physical activity is affected by gender norms.[141] There is pressure from society and from peers to appear and act feminine, and if they do too much exercise or the 'wrong' types of exercise (for example, rugby) they're seen as overly masculine. In general, the qualities encouraged in sports, such as competitiveness and strength, are at odds with stereotypical feminine ideals. Even for the girls who want to appear strong and capable, there is pressure to counterbalance these qualities to avoid being perceived as muscular or aggressive. Girls' relationship with exercise requires complex negotiations of gender roles, so it's not surprising that activity rates decline as they get older. That's where fitspo comes in, as people who post fitspo content are regularly 'normal' people (i.e. not celebrities or personal trainers) who advocate strength. These people can be positive role models for girls and young adults, and motivate them to keep being active by reassuring them that exercise doesn't negate their femininity. It goes at least some small way towards fighting extreme gender stereotypes, which is only a good thing.

Conclusion

The fitspo movement on Instagram, while seemingly having good intentions, may actually be causing more harm than good to a considerable part of the population by promoting one ideal image for what a 'fit and healthy' person looks like, and ultimately discourages people to exercise. Because of the image-focused nature of fitspo, it also (inadvertently or deliberately) encourages exercise for aesthetic and appearance purposes, which we know are linked to negative body image and disordered eating. There are so many great benefits to exercise, from blood cholesterol levels and feeling stronger and more able to improved mental health, stress management and the social aspect. Focusing on these positive outcomes generally means better self-esteem and body image, and therefore a lower risk of disordered eating and eating disorders. Focusing on aesthetics and making it about appearance likely means those mental health benefits don't happen. I want to encourage people to step away from seeing exercise as a means to manage weight, and instead think more like the 'This Girl Can' campaign, which aims to celebrate women's participation in sport regardless of physical appearance.

Around 50 per cent of adults who start an exercise programme drop out within the first six to twelve months, which shows how important it is to choose a form of movement that is enjoyable and sustainable. There's also no harm in trying something out, realising it's not suited, and trying something else instead.

Yes, in general people need to be encouraged to move their bodies and not be too sedentary, where possible. But it's not as simple as just 'move more'. To get all the amazingly positive benefits of exercise we need to focus away from weight loss, away from aesthetics, and recognise individuals at risk of overdoing it.

Quiz: Test your relationship with exercise

Please scale each of the following items.

	STRONGLY DISAGREE	SLIGHTLY DISAGREE	NEITHER AGREE NOR DISAGREE	SLIGHTLY AGREE	STRONGLY AGREE
Exercise is the most important thing in my life.	1	2	3	4	5
Conflicts have arisen between me and my family and/or my partner about the amount of exercise I do.	1	2	3	4	5
I use exercise as my main way of changing my mood.	1	2	3	4	5
I prioritise exercise over my work and social life.	1	2	3	4	5
If I have to miss an exercise session I feel moody and irritable.	1	2	3	4	5
If I cut down on the amount of exercise I do, and then start again, I always end up exercising as often as I did before.	1	2	3	4	5

The total score is categorised into 'asymptomatic' (scores 0–12), 'symptomatic' (13–23) and 'at risk' of exercise addiction (24 or greater).

This is not intended to diagnose but merely to highlight individuals who may be at risk so they can be aware and perhaps assess their behaviour and motivations for exercise.

Quiz: How do you feel about your body?

Please indicate whether each statement is true about you.

	NEVER	SELDOM	SOMETIMES	OFTEN	ALWAYS
I respect my body.	1	2	3	4	5
I feel good about my body.	1	2	3	4	5
I feel that my body has at least some good qualities.	1	2	3	4	5
I take a positive attitude towards my body.	1	2	3	4	5
I am attentive to my body's needs.	1	2	3	4	5
I feel love for my body.	1	2	3	4	5
I appreciate the different and unique characteristics of my body.	1	2	3	4	5
My behaviour reveals my positive attitude towards my body. For example, I hold my head high and smile.	1	2	3	4	5
I am comfortable in my body.	1	2	3	4	5
I feel like I am beautiful even if I am different from media images of attractive people (e.g. models/actors).	1	2	3	4	5

The higher your score, the greater an appreciation you have for your body. Add up your score and divide it by 10 to find your average. This isn't a diagnostic tool, more a guidance to see where you're at with your body image right now. The aim is to get your score higher, to averaging above 3, and if possible above 4.

9

HEALTH BEYOND NUTRITION

'*The causes of the causes are the social determinants of health and they influence not only lifestyle, but stress at work and at home, the environment, housing and transport.*'

MICHAEL MARMOT

If I asked you to draw a pie chart showing the different factors that affect our health, how many segments would there be? Which would be the largest?

I sampled one hundred random people on social media and asked them to do just this. Here is the amalgamation of their suggestions:

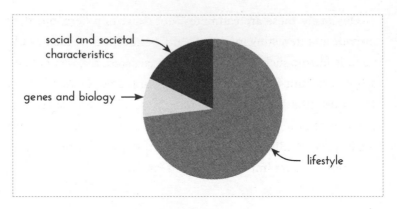

Figure 1. What people think determines population health

I think this is a pretty accurate representation of what our average person (who hasn't studied public health) thinks. A heavy emphasis on nutrition and exercise, with not many other factors getting a look in.

Compare this with the CDC* pie chart, which echoes WHO data.

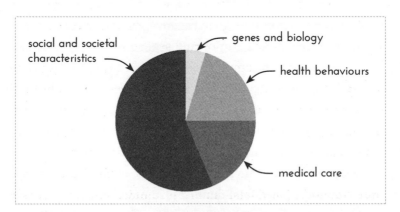

Figure 2. Actual determinants of population health

*   Centers for Disease Control and Prevention

Obviously these are estimates, not exact numbers, but they provide an interesting insight. Health behaviours – which would include factors such as nutrition, exercise, smoking, alcohol and so on – account for less than a quarter of the population health. The most significant variable here is socio-economic factors. Even within the 'health behaviours' category – the only one we really have significant control over – there are factors beyond nutrition that are important to address, such as sleep.

Sleep

How much sleep do you get, on average, a night? Is a good night's sleep a priority for you, or more of a luxury? Hopefully after reading this you'll realise just how important sleep is for our health.

During sleep, you cycle between periods of REM (rapid eye movement) and non-REM sleep, both of which are incredibly important and needed for good health. A typical sleep cycle takes around ninety minutes, so during a good night's sleep (seven to nine hours are recommended for adults) you'll go through around four to six cycles. You generally get more non-REM sleep earlier in the night, and more REM sleep closer to waking. During sleep, you're not just resting, your body works to restore your immune, nervous, skeletal and muscular systems.

Sleep is vital for our survival. We know this, because of a rare condition called fatal familial insomnia. Sufferers struggle with sleep, until over time they are unable to sleep at all. Life expectancy from that point onwards is a mere matter of months. There is no treatment.

There are two main factors that determine sleep: the circadian rhythm and adenosine. Our bodies have a natural circadian rhythm, which is set to around twenty-four hours. Not exactly twenty-four hours, but in that area. Seeing as a day is exactly twenty-four hours, this means the brain needs anchoring to essentially reset its internal clock back to exactly twenty-four hours each day. The best way to achieve this is through exposure to natural light. Social interactions and regular mealtimes can also help with this.

The brain communicates the cycle of day and night through releasing melatonin. This hormone is released into the bloodstream at night to signal that there is a lack of daylight and therefore it's time to sleep. It doesn't cause sleep, but signals to the body to begin the process of sleep and feeling sleepy.

Adenosine is released whenever you're awake, and builds up over the course of the day, resulting in sleep pressure. In the evenings, melatonin and adenosine are both high, which is why you feel most sleepy then. Adenosine is then broken down while you sleep so you feel refreshed when you wake up – unless you don't sleep for long enough and the breakdown process isn't complete. In that case you accumulate a 'sleep debt', which will build up until the adenosine is cleared. When you reach for your coffee first thing in the morning to wake you up, the caffeine blocks adenosine receptors so that adenosine can't bind, meaning your brain perceives there being less adenosine than is actually the case – and you feel less sleepy than you should! Once the caffeine is metabolised, you often experience a 'caffeine crash' as you're hit with all the adenosine that's been building up and hiding behind a wall of caffeine.

When it comes to food and sleep, it's recommended not to

eat too late as large meals just before bed are linked to reduced sleep quality. Ideally give yourself a good few hours between your last big meal and going to sleep. A small dessert or a snack if you're hungry won't have a big impact on your sleep quality; in fact, if you're hungry it's better to eat something as hunger will also prevent you from getting to sleep as easily.

Lack of sleep also has an impact on your food intake and food choices. When you're sleep-deprived (around six hours of sleep or less), your ghrelin levels increase while leptin decreases, so not only do you not get the normal 'I'm full' signals from leptin, but the 'I'm hungry' signal from ghrelin is amplified.[42] This means you'll feel hungrier than if you'd had a good night's sleep and are more likely to overeat. You're also more likely to reach for comfort foods, or more specifically, high-sugar, high-fat foods or salty snacks. Sleep deprivation is sometimes just a fact of life, and the occasional one-off isn't going to cause you many problems, but if you're regularly not getting enough sleep it disrupts your body's normal appetite hormone signalling, which makes it harder for you to be in tune with your body.

Alcohol, while appearing to help you get to sleep more easily, actually disrupts sleep. Alcohol has a sedative effect, which is a different state to sleep and more like anaesthesia. Alcohol affects sleep in two main ways: it fragments it so that you briefly awaken many times throughout the night (although it's highly likely you don't remember any of them) and it suppresses REM sleep.[142] This results in you not being as well rested as you'd expect, and having reduced memory function.

Overall, the effects of insufficient sleep are pretty damaging: depressed immune system, disruption of blood sugar levels, reduced concentration, impaired memory and increased risk of cancer, heart disease, stroke, dementia, depression and anxiety. Chronic sleep deprivation is also one of the major contributors to development of type 2 diabetes. In essence, shorter sleep time means a shorter lifespan.[143]

In the case of many of these diseases, but particularly heart disease, the effect of sleep deprivation is mediated by the fight-or-flight response. Sleep deprivation activates the sympathetic nervous system to the point where it's in overdrive, as well as increasing your body's cortisol level, which constricts your blood vessels, raising your blood pressure. Non-REM sleep, on the other hand, calms the sympathetic nervous system. You can really see this on a population level when the clocks change between GMT and BST. In spring, when the clocks move forward an hour, many people lose an hour of sleep and there is a spike in heart attacks the following day. In autumn, when the clocks move back and many people gain an hour of sleep, the opposite effect is observed, and we see a drop in heart attacks.[144] And that's the effect of just one hour of sleep.

I'm not saying all this to scare you, but just to give you that little push to make sleep more of a priority if you haven't already done so. For some bizarre reason, our society values and encourages sleep deprivation under the guise of being oh so busy and productive and always grinding. But you're far more likely to be productive, learn more, be healthier and be a nicer human being to those around you if you sleep well.

Quiz: Are you sleep-deprived?

IN THE LAST WEEK	YES/NO
Have you fallen asleep within 5 minutes? Or Has it taken you longer than an hour to get to sleep?	
Did you frequently wake up at night?	
Have you slept on average for 6 hours or less per night?	
Have you felt like you could fall asleep again before midday?	
Could you function relatively normally in the morning without coffee?	

The more questions you answered 'yes' to, the more likely it is that you're sleep-deprived. Hopefully I've convinced you that you should do something about that.

Stress

A quick reminder of the stress response: we respond to stress with a 'fight or flight' reaction, with our brains sending signals to our bodies via the HPA axis and the SAM system. The HPA axis increases adrenaline in the body and the SAM system increases cortisol, both hormones, both of which lead to a range of changes in different bodily systems. Acute stress can be beneficial and activate responses in the body that help you get through that stressful situation, whereas prolonged chronic stress leads to wear and tear on the body's regulatory systems. This can weaken any beneficial responses to stress, weaken the immune system and lead to increased risk of disease. The experience of chronic stress takes a serious toll on someone, both physically and psychologically.

Although we've been aware of a link between stress and health for a while, exactly how stress gets 'under your skin' and leads to poor health was mostly unknown. This is partly because scientists have only recently developed the necessary tools to look at the biological processes that link experiences of stress with disease.

Now we know that stress is linked to the onset of diseases such as heart disease, cancer and colds, as well as speeding up the process of ageing. We also know it's shown to aggravate conditions such as asthma, irritable bowel syndrome (IBS), arthritis, respiratory diseases, skin disorders and diabetes, and leads to symptoms such as headaches, muscular pain, stomach pain, insomnia and general tiredness.

The inflammatory response is an incredibly primitive mechanism in your body – elements of it existed even before the development of the nervous system. The stress response evolved from and is intricately linked to the inflammatory response, as stress can promote and encourage components of the immune system that are involved in inflammation. This means that stress hormones initiate an inflammatory response in the body. Almost all immune cells have receptors for one or more stress hormones.

Most people think of inflammation as the body's response to physical injury and infection, so when you get a cut or burn, for example, you'll notice the area feels warm and raised –

it's slightly inflamed. But inflammation also plays a role in several of the biggest diseases, thereby making inflammation a common link between stress and different conditions.

Stressors can enhance the risk of developing infectious disease, and they can also cause infectious illness episodes to hang around for longer, especially the common cold. I think we can all remember times where we were under stress, and then managed to catch a cold either during or just after a stressful experience. I know from my own experience that every year I would catch a bad cold a day or two after my university exams were finished. That's no coincidence. That anecdote is backed up by research. A cold that you catch when you're stressed often forces you to relax and spend some time resting. If you don't, the cold tends to last a lot longer and is harder to get rid of.

Stress, by activating the sympathetic nervous system and the HPA axis, causes the release of various stress hormones, which cause a higher heart rate and blood pressure, damage to artery wall linings, and an inflammatory response in the arteries. If this stress is repetitive or chronic, it can lead to atherosclerosis – a build-up of material in the arteries, potentially leading to blockage, which can trigger a heart attack or stroke.[145] Chronic life stress is now considered to be an important risk factor for heart disease, alongside diet and exercise.

Work-related stress is the most widely studied chronic life stress relative to heart disease. There are several aspects of the work environment that can play a role, one of them being job strain. Jobs with high demand but low autonomy and decision-making are more likely to lead to heart disease and related deaths. When work stress arises as a result of high demand and low reward, the risk of heart disease is high. Having lower job control also means higher risk of a heart attack. Taken together, all this strongly suggests that chronic stress, including work stress, can cause development of atherosclerosis and heart disease.[146]

This is just one example of a life stress that affects heart disease, but often stresses can cluster together, which further increases the risk of a heart attack or stroke. There is now abundant evidence that atherosclerosis is the end result of a chronic inflammatory process and that approximately 40–50 per cent of patients have no heart disease risk factors, just stress.

Stress can also play an important role in other conditions, such as diabetes. When under stress, blood sugar rises in response to cortisol release in order to supply energy for fight or flight – regardless of which one you end up doing, you're going to need extra energy. Cortisol inhibits insulin production in an attempt to prevent glucose from being stored, so instead it can be used immediately. If the stress is resolved quickly, cortisol drops, insulin goes up, and blood sugar levels go back to normal. But if the stress is chronic and cortisol is chronically high, this produces a state of insulin resistance, where the body's cells aren't as responsive to insulin. Over time, this can lead to type 2 diabetes.[147]

There have been some interesting insights recently that have suggested that stress-induced chronic inflammation may be a contributing factor in up to 15 per cent of all cancer cases.[148] The evidence tells us that stress itself doesn't directly cause cancer, but stressful situations can sometimes lead us to develop unhealthy habits, such as smoking or heavy drinking. We know that these things can lead to cancer (although not always), so in this way stress could indirectly increase cancer risk.

On a slightly less serious note than cancer and diabetes, many people experience some kind of gastrointestinal symptoms when stressed, such as stomach ache, diarrhoea or excess gas. This is because stress hormones slow the release of stomach acid and emptying of the stomach in preparation for fight or flight, and also speed up emptying of the colon – you don't want to focus on digestion if you're about to run away from a threat.

Weight stigma, which has been covered in Chapter 2, is a form of social stressor which can impact a person's health, as is racism or homophobia or any other form of discrimination. LGBTQ+ individuals are known to be at greater risk of mental health issues, and are more likely to seek mental health services compared with heterosexual people.[149] Discrimination and harassment also has a huge negative effect on the body image of transgender and non-binary folks.[150]

Ethnic minority groups that experience racism have higher rates of both mental and physical ill health, including heart disease, diabetes, anxiety and depression. This has been linked to over-activation of the HPA axis and chronic stress due to discrimination.[151]

Although stress is a strong risk factor for the various conditions mentioned, not everyone who experiences stress gets sick, so there must be individual differences that make some of us more likely to be affected by stress than others. Aside from the obvious genetics, we all have slightly different brains and slightly different neural pathways, and some of us have lower pain thresholds than others. We also have differently strong immune systems, which may play a role too. One important point is that stress is subjective, and affects some people more acutely and intensely than others. Some people have clear coping mechanisms in place or a robust support system that allows them to cope with stress more effectively than others. There is also some evidence that the way we perceive stress influences if, and how negatively, it affects us.

Some stress is good for us and is necessary. Positive stress is also known as eustress. It's motivating, exciting, manageable, improves performance and, most importantly, it's short-term. It's not chronic. A complete lack of stress is great if you're on holiday relaxing on a beach in the sunshine, but if you're trying to get a piece of work done, sit an exam or write a book (!), then having a little bit of stress in the form of a deadline, for example, can be highly motivating. A little stress helps focus the mind on the task at hand. But it depends on the person: if you're sitting in an exam and look up at the clock to see you have fifteen minutes left, you might think 'Fifteen minutes of focus. I can do this – just a few more things to write,' which is a positive injection of a little stress; or it could make you panic by causing a large stress response, which is unhelpful. At high levels of stress, performance and ability drops dramatically. We all have a different zone of optimal performance under stress, and knowing where you sit can help you focus better and avoid feeling overwhelmed.

Your mind is pretty damn powerful, and although a lot of the 'think yourself well' messages out there are bullshit, there is evidence that your beliefs can have quite a strong influence on your mood. If you believe that you have the ability and resources to handle a stressful situation, then it's far less likely to affect you negatively; whereas if you believe you can't handle it you're more likely to feel hopeless and out of control. This is a good thing, as while your emotions are hard to control and alter, you can change your thought patterns. If you are able to find a way to see your situation in a more positive light, you can alter your mood from negative to positive. This is exactly what I was illustrating in the example above about exams. Managing to cope with a stressful situation also gives us confidence that we can do it again.

If you believe you are able to have an impact and influence on events that affect your life, then you possess high levels of what is known as self-efficacy. This allows you to have a sense of control of stressful situations you encounter, so you're less likely to experience negative stress feelings. The perception of being in control is what's important, regardless of whether in reality you are or are not. The opposite is also true, so if you feel you aren't in control (even if you actually are), you will feel stressed. People may also feel out of control because they don't possess the appropriate coping skills to adequately cope with the situation.

Coping skills are tools that can be learned and carried around in your personal toolkit, on hand to help you cope with stressful situations. There are several popular approaches to reducing or managing stress that I want to mention, such as distraction techniques, pets, exercise and cognitive training.

Distraction

Some people find it incredibly helpful to distract their minds from stressful thoughts. Of course, this isn't possible in an acute stress situation such as an exam, but can be helpful if you're stressing about something unavoidable that's happening in the future, or something that you can't change. Popular distractions include doing chores, going to see friends, baking, watching a movie, games, art or books. It helps if the distraction is interesting and that you can immerse yourself in it, as it makes it easier to focus for long periods of time. In that sense, it is quite an individual thing.

Pets

Pets are so much less complicated than humans, and so our relationships with them are far more predictable. We know that if we feed a cat or dog and pay it attention, they will generally show us love in return. That consistency and predictability can be really comforting during a time when it feels like everything in life is spiralling out of control. There is also something satisfying and fulfilling about taking care of another living being, which positively influences our self-worth. Pets can also directly improve our mood, as they help us to feel less lonely and isolated, and therefore less stressed. In particular, walking a dog means going outside and the chance to interact with other people (pretty much everyone loves dogs). Stroking a cat or dog has direct physiological effects such as decreasing blood pressure, lowering heart rate and decreasing muscle tension, all of which helps us to feel less stressed.

Exercise

As we've already discussed in Chapter 8, moving your body is a great stress management tool. It focuses the mind, improves mood and releases endorphins. Yoga is believed to be particularly good for stress management due to its focus on breath work,

Quiz: How stressed are you?

Indicate how often you feel the way described in each of the following statements.

	NEVER	ALMOST NEVER	SOMETIMES	FAIRLY OFTEN	VERY OFTEN
I constantly feel tired or depleted.	1	2	3	4	5
I find myself over-reacting to little things.	1	2	3	4	5
I worry constantly.	1	2	3	4	5
I'm easily irritable.	1	2	3	4	5
I don't feel confident in my ability to cope with daily challenges.	1	2	3	4	5
When I'm stressed, I make unhealthy choices for myself.	1	2	3	4	5
My workplace feels like a high-stress environment.	1	2	3	4	5
I struggle to sleep at night because my mind is racing.	1	2	3	4	5

8-18 → low-stress lifestyle

19-27 → moderately stressed

28+ → high-stress lifestyle

meditation and the mind–body connection. A number of studies have shown that yoga may help reduce stress, as well as enhance mood and overall sense of well-being.[152]

Cognitive training

When we are stressed, we start to have more 'catastrophic' ways of thinking. Cognitive training or professional therapy services such as cognitive behavioural therapy (CBT) can help challenge and readdress these thoughts, rather than accepting them as truth. This technique is based not so much on preventing stress but more on changing how we perceive stress and respond to it when it arises so it becomes more manageable.

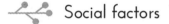 ## Social factors

Several lifestyle factors and environmental factors put us at risk of early death, such as smoking, physical inactivity, lack of sleep and air pollution. However, there is another key factor that is often overlooked, both in public health initiatives and in research, and that is social factors.

In countries like the UK, the quality and quantity of social relationships is decreasing. We have fewer friends than before, and even fewer who we see regularly in person rather than just online. This has been blamed on a number of reasons, including reduced intergenerational living, ease of movement, delayed marriage, larger numbers of single-parent households and more people choosing to live alone. Despite the huge amount of online connection we now have with other people, overall this doesn't seem to have had a positive effect on our social connections. Perhaps it has made us lazy? It is more common now for people to report feeling lonely despite being surrounded by hundreds or thousands of virtual 'friends' and profiles. People are becoming increasingly more socially isolated. Given these trends, it's vital that we are all aware of the significance of our social relationships and the impact they have on our health.

Living alone and not having regular social contact are all signs of social isolation. Loneliness is a subjective state; it's the perception of social isolation or the subjective experience of being lonely. But loneliness and social isolation are not the same thing. For instance, someone may be socially isolated but perfectly content with being in that situation, whereas someone else may have frequent contact with friends but still feel lonely as it's not enough for them.

Data from seventy studies with over three million participants showed that social isolation and loneliness result in higher risk of early death. People who are lonely and socially isolated are around 30 per cent more likely to die earlier.[153] It isn't something limited to elderly people either, but all adults of all ages.

Combining the effects of 148 studies shows that our experiences within social relationships significantly predict mortality. We are 50 per cent more likely to survive any given year if we have good relationships with friends and/or family.[154] This is regardless of age, sex and cause of death. This has about the same effect on your life as quitting smoking, and has a greater effect than weight and physical inactivity, so it's pretty significant overall.

People with active social lives recover faster from illness, are more likely to comply with medication, and have shorter hospital stays.[155] They are also less likely to become ill in the first place, with lower risk of heart attack, stroke, dementia and other diseases.

The reasons that social relationships lead to better health overall are complex, as they influence healthy behaviours but also have a more direct effect on health by affecting biochemical changes in our bodies, which then affect disease outcomes. One big example is that there is a strong link between social support and having a stronger, more resilient immune system.[154]

There is a clear link between social isolation and reduced psychological well-being. Smaller social networks, fewer close relationships and inadequate social support have all been linked to depression.[156] But it's difficult to be sure how much of that comes from social isolation, compared to personality traits such as being an introvert, which mean people don't want to participate in a lot of social situations and prefer to be alone. Cutting yourself off from friends and family can also occur as a result of depression and not wishing to be a burden on others, even though this tends to make the depression worse.

Having social connections is not just important for psychological and emotional well-being, but also physical health. There are two pathways that are suggested to influence health. One involves behavioural processes such as health behaviours. The idea is that social support promotes health, as it encourages healthier behaviours such as exercise, eating a balanced diet, sleeping well and not smoking. But that is only part of the story, as it's also possible for social interactions to encourage negative health behaviours such as excessive alcohol consumption or staying up way too late and not getting enough sleep. The other pathway involves psychological processes such as mood and emotions and feelings of control. For example, having social support from friends can make stressful life experiences feel less overwhelming and more manageable. This effect applies to both mental and physical health outcomes.

An example of how this manifests in disease is that being around friends reduces your blood pressure,[157] which reduces your risk of heart disease. There is also evidence that social relationships lead to lower adrenaline and cortisol levels – both important stress hormones – which means a stronger immune system that isn't suppressed by stress. Another important hormone is oxytocin, sometimes known as the love hormone. This is the hormone that is released during breastfeeding, when you give someone a hug, and during sex. It's an important hormone for human bonding, as it encourages trust and understanding through being able to read people's emotional facial expressions.

Some researchers look at social bonds from a more evolutionary perspective, suggesting that humans are fundamentally motivated to maintain a social network because of the protection and support that others provide. It allows us to not have to worry about certain things in life as we can delegate them to others we trust. Because of this, cutting social ties can be particularly distressing to us, whether it's a break-up, loss of a friend, or divorce. Humans have a basic need to belong and to be social; it seems to be ingrained in our evolutionary history and genetic make-up.

This goes some way towards explaining why people who are more socially connected with family and friends are happier, and live longer, healthier lives with fewer physical and mental health problems than people who are less socially connected. Being born into a close family means a child is given the best social start in life, by laying the foundations of feeling loved and valued. It also allows them to learn to build supportive relationships; develop intellectual, social and emotional skills; and develop lifelong healthy habits. Family ties in adulthood, such as having a strong, healthy, loving relationship with a partner, has positive impacts on health and provides us with support to deal with life's challenges. We know that being part of a social network (in person, not online) gives people meaningful roles that provide self-esteem and give a sense of purpose. That could be something as simple as carrying the responsibility of organising a monthly dinner party, or attending a theatre group where each person has a different role to play. Take that away from someone and it can affect their self-worth and happiness.

Interestingly, having a few close friends is important to all adults, but having close family ties is more important to men than women for their well-being.[158]

Healthcare professionals, teachers, the media and the general public all take smoking, nutrition and exercise seriously, but often neglect social relationships. We need to take social health into account as well as physical and mental health, if we want to get an overall picture of someone.

Quiz: How lonely are you?

Indicate how often you feel the way described in each of the following statements.

	NEVER	RARELY	SOMETIMES	OFTEN
I feel in tune with the people around me.	4	3	2	1
I lack companionship.	1	2	3	4
There is no one I can turn to.	1	2	3	4
I do not feel alone.	4	3	2	1
I feel part of a group of friends.	4	3	2	1
I have a lot in common with the people around me.	4	3	2	1
I am no longer close to anyone.	1	2	3	4
My interests and ideas are not shared by those around me.	1	2	3	4
I am an outgoing person.	4	3	2	1
There are people I feel close to.	4	3	2	1
I feel left out.	1	2	3	4
My social relationships are superficial.	1	2	3	4
No one really knows me well.	1	2	3	4
I feel isolated from others.	1	2	3	4
I can find companionship when I want it.	4	3	2	1

	NEVER	RARELY	SOMETIMES	OFTEN
There are people who really understand me.	4	3	2	1
I am unhappy being so withdrawn.	1	2	3	4
People are around me but not with me.	1	2	3	4
There are people I can talk to.	4	3	2	1
There are people I can turn to.	4	3	2	1

The higher the score, the more lonely it seems you are.

Healthcare/medical care

It probably goes without saying that access to healthcare usually means better health. Equal access to healthcare has been a central focus in the NHS since its inception in 1948. In theory, there shouldn't be discrepancies in access to healthcare, as the NHS is free to patients at the point of use, but that isn't the case. Health needs will not be the same across different areas of the country and will vary according to the socio-economic characteristics of an area. There are a few reasons why there are variations from region to region when it comes to access to healthcare: some health services may not be available to certain population groups – for example, child and adolescent mental health services, or IVF clinics. The quality of services may also vary, as different practitioners will have varying degrees of expertise and interests. Equal access doesn't necessarily mean equal treatment. There may also be discrepancies in patients' awareness about the services available, and there can be additional costs, such as for prescriptions.[159]

When a medical appointment is booked, a patient generally has to physically get to the clinic or facility (with the exception of phone consultations, for example). Geography, local support and access to transport all influence how easily someone can attend an appointment. The cost of transport and distance to the GP surgery can also be a factor. Almost 40 per cent of people living in rural areas do not have a GP within 2 km, compared with only 1 per cent in urban areas. Older people are particularly susceptible to these factors, as are people with families, since family commitments can take priority, which affects whether a patient is free to attend an appointment or be brought to an appointment by another person. People working regular daytime hours may not be able to take time off work for appointments, and working parents may not be able to take time off to take their children to an appointment. Extended opening hours in some GP surgeries have definitely helped with this, but only up to a point.

Access to mental healthcare is a particularly large problem, with waiting times steadily increasing, and patients sometimes having to be sent across the country – sometimes from Oxford all the way to Scotland – for intensive psychiatric care. It probably goes without saying that this can have a huge effect on recovery if patients are unable to see family as often, and places an extra time and cost burden on family and friends to afford travel.

Although health in urban areas in general is usually worse than in rural areas, countryside living does come with the disadvantage of more difficult access to GP and hospital care.[160]

As an example, if you needed joint surgery, the probability of getting it depends on who you are and where you live. In particular, older people, women, and those living in deprived areas seemed to be disadvantaged.[161] That's not equal access.

Of course, the UK is very fortunate to have a healthcare system that is free at the point of access. In countries without a national health service, such as the US, insurance policies determine access to and affordability of healthcare, and lack of insurance is an additional risk. The US healthcare system is not a universally accessible system - it is a publicly and privately funded mixture of systems and programmes. Insured Americans are covered by both public and private health insurance, with the majority covered by insurance plans through their employers. Government-funded programmes, such as Medicaid and Medicare, also provide healthcare coverage to some vulnerable population groups. The US has excellent healthcare facilities, but not everyone, especially those who are uninsured, can afford to access these. The primary reason Americans give for problems accessing healthcare is the prohibitively high cost. In fact, for a patient who has no insurance, a medical bill can lead to lifelong debt.

In Australia, for example, all permanent Australian residents have access to Medicare, the state healthcare provider, and this is paid for through taxes. While most of the time an Australian will never see the bill for their medical care, sometimes they'll have to pay and then claim back the money, which can put someone in financial difficulty. The government is also trying to persuade anyone who earns enough to take out private policies on top of their state coverage to relieve pressure on the public system. On the one hand, this makes sense, as it leaves the public system more available to those who can't afford private insurance; but it also creates a divide between those who have private healthcare and those who don't, with differences in accessibility to health services. For example, if you have private insurance you can be treated at both public and private hospitals – more choice – whereas if you don't you can only be treated at public hospitals.

Because of the vastly different healthcare systems around the world, the notion of the word 'access' is dependent on context. In the US, access usually means whether the individual is insured, and if so, to what degree. In Europe, however, access is more likely to mean how easy it is for a patient to secure particular services, at a certain level of quality, and whether there are any personal inconveniences such as waiting times or distances to travel.

Socio-economic factors

If I asked you 'What causes poor health and disease?', you might say poor diet and lack of exercise. And you'd be right, to an extent. But what causes poor diet? What is the cause of the cause? These are the very sources of the problems of health we face in society, and they are the social determinants of health.

Social determinants of health refer to the social, cultural, political, economic, commercial and environmental factors that shape the conditions in which we are born, live and work. They are also sometimes referred to as the wider determinants of health, or socio-economic factors.

I really like the 'rainbow' model of the determinants of health, as it illustrates this in the form of multiple layers of influence, one on top of the other. At the centre we have our own individual actions, and on top of that are layered influences of family, friends, community and neighbourhoods. On top of that are the social and economic structures such as employment and housing, and finally on top of that there are national policies on welfare as well as cultural influences, such as the role of women. Each layer is influenced and affected by the layer above it.

We see weight as purely dictated by lifestyle choices, primarily diet and exercise, but what about factors that are beyond our control? What always gets left out of the conversation on the 'war on obesity' is the huge disparity between high- and low-income families.

For starters, the life expectancy difference between the most and the least deprived areas is nine years for males and seven years for females. The UK is a wealthy society, yet a baby girl born in Richmond upon Thames can expect to live seven years longer, and live seventeen more years in good health, compared with a baby girl born in Manchester. There's a reason we call it the North–South divide. In general, the lower an individual's social position, the poorer their health is likely to be.[162]

These social determinants, or causes of causes, can influence our health in many ways, including through our health behaviours such as food choice and exercise. But our own individual control over these behaviours is often limited, as any unhealthy behaviours are usually not the definitive cause of poor health, but are at the end point of a long chain of cause and effect in people's lives. If you're struggling with this concept I'd like to gently remind you of a great quote I've seen online: 'If you don't have to think about it, it's a privilege.' Saying someone has privilege is not a moral judgement. Becoming aware of your privilege shouldn't be a source of guilt, although it's natural for the thought to come with defensive feelings, but should be seen as an opportunity to learn. For example, I recognise that I have white privilege, thin privilege, educational privilege and financial privilege as I grew up in a middle-class family. Acknowledging this is the first step to understanding that someone else might not have had the same experiences in life. Having a higher income comes with a great deal of privilege, and can lead us to believe that all our health behaviours, particularly our food choices, are perfectly within our control, because we have no financial barriers that prevent us from eating the way we want to. If you don't struggle to afford eating a varied balanced diet, if you have no financial barrier, no education barrier, no time barrier, then you are in an incredibly privileged position. That's not a criticism, but something to think about as you read the rest of this section.

There are several of these 'causes of causes' that I want to highlight: education, employment, housing, our surroundings, and money/income.

Education

Level of education is strongly linked with health. The more educated someone is, the less likely they are to suffer from chronic conditions, suffer from mental health issues such as depression or anxiety, or consider themselves to be in poor health.[163] Education impacts on many areas in life such as quality of work, future income, involvement in crime and risk of premature death. A good education can help access to good work, problem-solving, feeling valued and empowered, and supportive social connections. These all help people to live longer, healthier lives by increasing opportunities and limiting exposure to some of life's challenges.

Education is also affected by income. In 2015 to 2016, 14 per cent of children in England were eligible for free school meals, which are only available to those who come from low-income households. These children were significantly less likely to reach a good level of physical, personal, social and emotional development than children not eligible for free school meals. This means that children from more deprived areas are less likely to receive a good education, which means they are more at risk of long-term health conditions and less likely to be able to live long, healthy lives.

Employment

Employment is one of the most important determinants of health, as it is closely related to income. Being unemployed puts someone at greater risk of poor health and early death. Young people in particular who are not in employment, education or training are at greater risk of poor physical and mental health, as well as being more likely to have lower quality jobs later, with lower income.[164]

The effect of unemployment goes beyond just the individual. Children growing up in households where both parents are unemployed are almost twice as likely to fail at all stages of education compared with children growing up in families where at least one parent is working.

As with education, there is a clear social gradient when it comes to unemployment. Unemployment in the most deprived areas is considerably higher than in the least deprived areas. So how does this affect health? Good working conditions, working in a safe environment, practices that protect employees' well-being, good pay... These factors all create an environment where employees are more supported, have opportunities to grow and progress, and feel a sense of autonomy over their work. Being in that kind of environment will be much less taxing on stress and mental health in particular than a working environment with poor conditions, chance of injury or contact with harmful toxic substances.[165] Lower-paid employment is more likely to have higher risk of injury and low levels of job control – which can include monotony, no sick pay and only being allowed breaks at highly specific times. Good work provides people with the opportunity to afford basic living standards, to be able to participate in the community and have a social life, as well as feel a sense of identity, self-esteem and purpose.

Our mental well-being is particularly affected by unemployment. Loss of income is the obvious culprit, but there are more nuanced factors at play. For many people, their job is what gets them out of bed in the morning, adds structure to their day and makes them feel like they have a sense of purpose and self-worth. A job is where they make connections and friends, and feel a sense of achievement. All this is taken away with unemployment.

In the longer term, unemployment, poverty and psychological issues can become a vicious circle. Being unemployed and poor can lead to poorer health outcomes, which in turn hinders someone's attempts to escape unemployment and poverty. Unemployment often happens in repeated spells: once one job is lost, the next is often less secure.[166]

Housing

A house is more than just a roof over our heads: it's our home, where we grow up or grow old, where we are supposed to feel safe and comfortable and warm.

Fuel poverty is described as being when a household cannot afford to keep adequately warm at a reasonable cost, which again relates back to income. Children living in cold homes are more than twice as likely to suffer from respiratory problems as children living in warm homes.[167] Living conditions that are damp and mouldy also increase the likelihood of health problems including wheeze and other respiratory problems, aches and pains, diarrhoea, headaches and fever.

Overcrowding is another issue, as this has particularly negative effects on mental health, as well as being thought to increase vulnerability to airborne infections, diarrhoea and coughs.[168]

Surroundings

Our health is influenced by our surroundings – how they make us feel and the opportunities they provide. This can include the public transport systems that allow us to get to work, being near shops and schools to make it easier to walk to them, and having green spaces for play. The latter is particularly important, as having well-maintained and easy-to-reach green spaces makes it easier for people to be physically active.[169] Public open spaces in higher socio-economic areas are more likely to have trees, ponds, walking and cycling paths and picnic tables. These are all features that encourage being outdoors and promote physical activity for both children and adults.[170] Green spaces in general, regardless of their facilities, are more available to higher income neighbourhoods. Plus there are issues of crime and traffic, neither of which make it easier for children to play outside.

Urban areas in general, particularly big cities, have lower air quality than rural areas, which affects health. People living in the most income-deprived neighbourhoods may be most exposed to air pollution, which affects risk of respiratory diseases as well as early death.[171]

In 2014, Transport for London adopted an action plan to improve air quality, reduce congestion and create healthy surroundings for people to live, work, travel and play. A healthy street is one that has things to do, places to rest, shelter and clean air. It has to feel safe and not be too noisy. It's an environment where people are happy to live and to walk around. All these things make for positive surroundings that positively affect our health.

Money/income

This is the big one! A lot of the previous aspects of socio-economics come back to money/income. There is a strong association between income and health, and many aspects of health improve as income increases. Beyond that, income also has an effect on others – for example, your parents' income will have affected your early development, your education, and therefore your employment and income.

In simple terms, not having enough income can lead to poor health because it makes it more difficult to avoid stress, it fosters a feeling of being out of control, you don't have a financial safety net, and certain resources and experiences will be out of reach. Money can enable people to access the support and services they need to participate fully in society. Limited income or access to fresh fruits and vegetables can make it more difficult for people to adopt healthier lifestyle choices.[172] Time is money, and having more money usually means having more time – time for things like chopping vegetables, making soup, slow-cooking and food shopping. A tired working parent who arrives home in the evening to hungry children may have neither the energy nor the time to spend half an hour preparing a meal. Having a higher income also means that trying new recipes and ingredients carries fewer risks, especially with children, as if they don't like it and won't eat it you can just make or buy something else instead.

There are two explanations for why money and income are linked to health. The first is that living on very little income is stressful, and as we have seen, stress has huge, far-reaching impacts on health. The second is that people feel of lower status in society compared with others, because of the lack of income, and that causes distress. These negative feelings and sensations can cause real biochemical changes in the body, which over time can wear down the immune system and other bodily functions. It's also important to point out that these negative feelings and distress lead to mental health problems being more prevalent among disadvantaged groups. The stress of experiencing racism or homophobia regularly, the stress of weight stigma, and the stress of constantly having to worry about money can all lead to mental health issues such as depression or anxiety. Some people may use unhealthy behaviours such as smoking or drinking alcohol as a method of coping with the stress they are under. Healthy behaviours can be expensive – for example, joining a gym or taking part in school sports clubs. It's also important to note that these stresses may mean someone focuses more on the present at the expense of the future, because the future is uncertain; and so someone might be less concerned with the long-term, health-damaging effects of behaviours that bring them pleasure or stress relief in the present moment.

Sometimes the simple arguments make sense – for example, that low income leads to lower quality diet, which has negative health consequences. But it's also a little bit more complicated than that. There is a web of complex factors that link socio-economic factors to health. For example, low income can lead to stress, which leads to depression, which discourages exercise, which can lead to poorer health. Or low income can lead someone to pick up an extra job with low autonomy, which is stressful, which causes negative emotions and distress, which over time affects the immune system and cardiovascular system and increases risk of infection and heart disease. It's complex.

Having a higher income generally means being able to afford to live in a more affluent area, which comes with better air quality, better facilities, better access to healthcare, higher density of exercise studios (the more middle class an area is, the more yoga studios pop up) and better schools. All these things carry health benefits.

Money and income affect so many different aspects of health, and affect us throughout our lives, from birth to childhood education, to employment, and into retirement. Income from employment is affected by education, which in turn is affected by childhood health and parental income.[173] This means that the relationship between money and health is intergenerational and bidirectional: for example, parents' income influences their children's health, and children's health influences their later earning capacity and their future income.

Let's relate this back to weight

Hopefully, it's now clear that all these factors are interlinked, and money is a key part of that. Although people are living longer now than ever before, it still remains that those in socially disadvantaged groups are more likely to face conditions that lead to poorer health and an earlier death. These health inequalities don't just exist between the very rich and the very poor in society – they span the entire population.

Bringing this back to weight and health for a moment, research investigating socio-economic disparities in weight have shown that factors outside our immediate control – such as income, neighbourhood, ethnicity, gender and level of education – all influence weight. Individuals who are marginalised either through low socio-economic status and/or non-white ethnicity are more likely to be in larger bodies, due to stress and these social determinants of health.[174] Looking at weight through a larger intersectional lens, those who are most disadvantaged – particularly if in more than one area (e.g. low income and ethnic minority group) – are more likely to be fat, and there is a gradient across the spectrum of wealth rather than simply a rich–poor divide. While those in the best socio-economic position tend to have the best health and those in the worst circumstances the poorest health, for those in between, small changes in income or other socio-economic factors can have an impact on health risk, as each slight improvement in position improves health. For example, there seems to be a lower risk of early death among people who have higher degrees compared with standard degrees[175], which suggests a continuous gradient in health rather than a large step up between groups. Income often displays a continuous gradient with health. At some point there may no longer be any health gains from more income, but for the vast majority of people it really does make a difference.

What do I want you to take away from this? First, hopefully this has shown you that health is so much more than just what we eat, and there are real and distinct barriers that prevent people from having control over their health. What we eat and how we move our body isn't purely down to individual choice; we only tend to think that way if we've never experienced those barriers for ourselves. But they are there, and we need to acknowledge them, and use them to remind ourselves that we can't judge and shouldn't shame ourselves or other people for the food choices they make. It's not that simple. We need compassion and understanding to improve population health, not stigma and stress.

10

WHAT REALLY IS
HEALTHY?

Over the course of this book, we've examined a whole bunch of different ways in which our perception and ideas about health can be misguided. But I want to end this book on a positive note, because it's not all doom and gloom. It's not as though we're all destined for poor mental and physical health. And yes, we can absolutely look after one without negatively impacting the other.

So here are my solutions and recommendations for how to tackle each of the issues outlined in the different chapters. What can you do to help improve your health? A great deal, it turns out.

Health gain, not weight loss

As we've seen from the chapter on weight and health, focusing on weight loss, which has been the primary focus so far, hasn't worked and hasn't been helpful. It stigmatises fat bodies, and it ignores thin bodies who are engaging in unhealthy behaviours and gives them a free pass simply because of the way they look.

Focusing on four key health-promoting behaviours – eating fruits and vegetables, exercising, not smoking, and moderate drinking – provides health benefits to everyone, regardless of their shape or size. These are the kinds of messages we need – messages that are health-focused, non-stigmatising and inclusive of everyone.

But if you're not going on a diet, then what? What's the alternative?

When it comes to health, there is no one simple solution. Anyone who says so is lying or has a very specific agenda (which usually makes them a lot of money). I want to offer you one possible solution. Not THE solution. Simply A solution. One I use in clinic that I find ethical, compassionate and effective.

Intuitive eating is a model developed by two dietitians in the US, Evelyn Tribole and Elyse Resch. Intuitive eating is an intervention and tool to help people move away from diet plans, food rules and so on, and instead learn to trust their internal signals of physical hunger and fullness. There are ten principles that underpin this, which include rejecting the diet mentality, honouring hunger and fullness, challenging unhelpful food thoughts, making peace with all foods, and rediscovering the joy in food.

Intuitive eating is not simply eating whatever you want whenever you want. It's more nuanced than that. The idea is based on how we ate as babies. Our parents might dictate our mealtimes for us, but we were in charge of how much we ate, and to a certain extent in charge of what we ate. Babies will happily eat and eat, then turn their heads away and throw things when they're done. Their bodies tell them when they've had enough, not a calorie counter and not a diet plan. We are all able to regulate how much we need to eat and when, without relying on external factors.

That doesn't mean it's easy. If you've spent years and years on various diets that have given you a strict set of rules about what, when and how much you can eat, you can't undo that overnight. If you've been in a restrictive mode for a while, your body might not even produce the proper hunger signals any more, although they absolutely come back with time.

What often happens when clients start to reject the diet mentality is that they do a total one-eighty and start eating everything that was 'forbidden' to them on whatever diet(s) they were on. They go nuts on biscuits and cake and ice cream and chocolate and pizza and bread ... and they feel scared and out of control. This can then trigger restriction and dieting behaviour again, which is why I recommend seeking professional guidance if you feel overwhelmed at the thought of rejecting dieting.

This is why intuitive eating has a little more structure to it, and why I start by getting an understanding of someone's dieting history and seeing where their hunger cues are at. It's baby steps. Start by getting to know your hunger signals that your body is sending you. Imagine your hunger and fullness like a fuel gauge, where zero or empty is so hungry you might pass out, and full or ten is so full you feel like you might explode. Think Christmas dinner plus mince pies plus cheese plus wine. A proper food coma. You want to recognise what comfortable hunger and comfortable fullness feel like to you, and use this to start guiding you on when and how much to eat. Don't think of it as a rule – here there are no rules. But it's a guideline.

Awareness on its own isn't enough, though – you need to act on it. Once you're more able to recognise and respond to your hunger signals, I then move on to looking at food rules. A key part of the intuitive eating process is being ok and comfortable with ALL foods. Even the scary ones. Especially the scary ones. This is known as unconditional permission to eat, and it's a gradual process. Start with one scary food, and eat it whenever you feel like. You might at this point end up eating a lot of it, which is fine. You've been in a deprivation mindset for so long that food becomes so special, so exciting, that you can't get enough of it; and your body is scared that you'll start restricting again, and in the back of your mind there's often still that mentality of 'If I don't eat it now, I don't know when I'll be able to have it again'... This is a 'last supper' mentality, and you eat like it's your last meal on earth. Understandably this is a bit scary, and plenty of clients worry that they're not eating healthily enough, or they're going to gain weight. But I promise this calms down after a while, as eventually you can get bored with anything if you eat it enough. If you were to eat ice cream for breakfast, lunch and dinner, I bet it wouldn't take long for you to desperately start craving something different. For some people it might take less than a day, for others a few days.

Over time, your body starts to realise that you're not going back on a diet again, and you can eat these foods whenever you want. Generally, this makes them boring, especially when they're easily accessible. We always want what we can't have; so if you can eat a doughnut every day, you might at first, but then one day you might decide 'Nope, I don't feel like it today', and you calmly say no because you know tomorrow is another day where you can have a doughnut if you want it.

This goes completely against what I see a lot of doctors advising, which is if you don't feel in control around it, don't have it in the house. While I can understand this 'out of sight, out of mind' logic, I don't think it's sustainable. What happens when you are then exposed to those foods, perhaps at a friend's house or on holiday? You're going to face-plant straight into it and then feel guilty. And so, while I know my way of looking at this seems unconventional and harder, it also works far better long term, and without the feelings of guilt and shame. I don't think it's enough to just focus on having a healthy body; you need a healthy mind too, and that includes how you think and feel about food. A healthy relationship with food doesn't include guilt and shame.

Alongside all this work on reframing ideas and perceptions around food comes body-image work, self-care and self-compassion, but you'll have to keep reading to find out more about those. In the end, what I share here can't replace having weekly consultations with me. But I hope I've piqued your interest, and if you're looking to find out more about the intuitive eating approach, I recommend two books: *Intuitive Eating* by Tribole and Resch; and *Just Eat It* by Laura Thomas. They go into far more detail about this than I am sharing here, as to do justice to the approach requires a whole other book in itself.

The biggest question people ask about intuitive eating is, 'Will I lose weight?' Maybe, but that's not the point. Intuitive eating isn't a weight-loss tool. The whole point of it is to put weight loss on the back burner and focus on your overall health. You may lose weight, you may not, but the idea is that you'll reach your set-point (what your brain thinks is healthiest) weight that your body is comfortable at, and you'll have learned amazing skills for life that don't depend on any person, plan or rule but your own body. It's not about perfection; it's about working with your body rather than fighting it, feeling comfortable in your body, and enjoying everything life has to offer, including food.

A note for all the female-identifying or non-binary folks out there: I like to think of rejecting diet culture as a feminist stance to take. Our patriarchal society has gone to great lengths to suppress us through diets, because if we're so focused on how small we are and how pretty we have to be to please men, it leaves us with far less headspace to be fierce, strong, independent people who can change the world. The research backs this up – when researchers asked women to take a maths test while wearing a swimsuit, they performed badly.[176] Diet culture literally robs us of our ability to think properly, through body shame and self-objectification. Get angry, get really mad about this, read about it (I highly recommend starting with Naomi Wolf's *The Beauty Myth*), and take a stand by not being complicit with diet culture.

And to all the men, particularly the cis-het men out there: diet culture tells you that you aren't manly enough if you don't look the way they want you to. This affects you too, and it affects all the women in your life in particular. So be a feminist and an ally.

For me, a non-diet approach is the best, most evidence-based and ethical approach to helping improve people's health. It has support from an increasing number of studies, it takes the individual's experience into consideration and is tailored to them, it's compassionate and kind, and it's non-stigmatising. It's a breath of fresh air in this world polluted with diet culture.

Emotional eating

Many online articles will say things like 'Emotional hunger can't be filled with food,' 'You feel worse after emotional eating,' and 'How to put a stop to emotional eating,' but these ideas are all wrong. You CAN fill emotional hunger with food, you can feel better after emotional eating, and you don't need to put a complete stop to it. It's ok to have emotional eating as part of your coping mechanisms, but it shouldn't be the only tool you have.

Emotional eating is a powerful and effective way to find temporary relief from many of life's challenges. If it didn't work so well, we wouldn't all be doing it.

Many of us believe that we eat our feelings. We're very open about that, and so we reprimand ourselves and tell ourselves we need some self-control and to get a grip. That's not a kind or helpful message to give ourselves.

Identifying hunger and fullness is one of the key aspects of learning intuitive eating. Once you're more aware of your hunger and fullness, this can help with emotional eating as well. Not only does it help you identify if you're actually physically hungry; with practice it also becomes a tool to help you stop and think for a moment, and stop the cycle of automatically reaching for food in response to emotions.

If you're getting to the point where you're so hungry you could eat the entire contents of the fridge in one go, it's worth reassessing your eating habits to try and avoid this as much as possible. It won't work one hundred per cent of the time – that's just life – but preventing this level of hunger is a great way to feel more in control and more comfortable about your eating. Often when we're that hungry we eat a lot, and we eat it quickly, and twenty minutes later we realise 'Oh God, I'm so full'. Cue feelings of guilt and shame. You end up going from intense hunger to intense fullness without really feeling any of the nuance of in between. Avoiding these extremes of hunger and fullness, where possible has three great benefits. First, it allows you to be more aware of how you're feeling as you eat, and prevents swinging from extreme hunger to extreme fullness. Second, it means you're less likely to feel guilt and shame, which are horrible negative emotions around food. Third, you feel more comfortable in your body, as you're generally staying within manageable hunger and comfortable, contented fullness, rather than feeling pain.

Recognising if you're physically or emotionally hungry is the first step. So you've recognised you're actually physically hungry: great, go and eat something. Or you've realised you're emotionally hungry – what do you do next?

Identify your triggers

Try to recognise what emotion it is you're feeling. What led you to feel that way? If you're finding it hard to think it through in your own mind, writing it down or talking it through with someone can be incredibly helpful. There's something about verbalising your thoughts that makes them more concrete, more real, and helps you process them without it being a jumbled mess in your head. We talked through the most common emotions that generally lead to emotional eating in Chapter 3, but here's a handy word cloud to get you started:

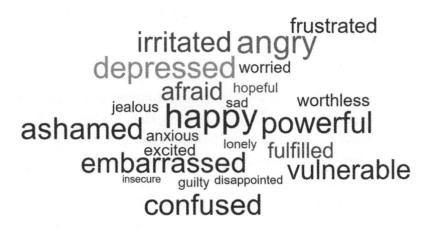

Satisfy your needs

Eating your emotions feels comfortable as it means we don't have to deal with them, so in the short term it can feel like the ideal solution. Remember that emotional eating in itself is not a problem. As far as coping mechanisms go, it's definitely far better than taking drugs or getting blind drunk. But ideally food shouldn't be the only thing that helps you deal with emotions.

Some other things that could help you out are:

- Cuddling a pet
- Calling a friend or family member

- Having a hot, relaxing bath with candles and music
- Going for a run or a yoga class
- Reading a book
- Painting your nails
- Watching a sad movie you know will help you cry (if that's what you need)
- Therapy

This is by no means an exhaustive list but will hopefully give you some ideas to find out what's in your emotional toolkit. Also, the idea isn't that these things completely replace emotional eating, but rather work alongside it – for example, eating chocolate in the bath or ice cream while watching a movie. It's unrealistic to remove emotional eating entirely. We aren't robots; we all have emotional connections to food, and they're part of what makes us wonderfully human.

Mindful eating

In essence, mindful eating involves a greater awareness of what you're eating, savouring it in a non-judgemental way, and hopefully enjoying your food more. It's not a tool to control what you eat, and I don't want you to see it as a weight-loss tool. There's an assumption that by eating mindfully you'll end up eating less, and for some people that might be the case, but that's not a guarantee. It's also not the point of mindful eating. It can help you work out the right amount of food for you on that day, in that meal, in that specific instance. That amount will vary with each day and each meal, depending on a whole host of factors.

If you're interested in mindfulness as a practice, there are some wonderful resources and books available. Here I want to simply give you a brief introduction to help you eat more mindfully. Often we find ourselves eating at our desks at work or in front of the TV, which distracts us from our food. Now what I don't want is for you to think you can never do this, because that's unrealistic and it's a food rule, which I hate. But if you can commit to having just one meal a day or a few meals a week where you commit yourself to eating mindfully, that is more than enough.

Before you eat, remove any distractions and make sure you're nice and relaxed. Close your eyes and be aware of how your body feels. Try to go beyond just 'hungry' and think about where the hunger is and what it feels like. Look at your food – what looks appealing about it? How does it smell? Take a bite and savour it in your mouth. Think about the flavours. Swallow, and take another mouthful, each time being aware of the flavours in your mouth. After about five minutes or so, stop and assess how your body feels. Then carry on. Once you've finished eating, try to articulate exactly what was enjoyable about that meal. How do you feel now? Did the meal fully satisfy you? If not, why not? What was missing?

You may find that the food was far more delicious by eating it this way. Or you may find that a food you thought you liked actually isn't that tasty after all. Your tastes can change over time. For example, I thought I loved broccoli, and when I used this technique recently I discovered that unless it's smothered in pesto or hummus I'm not such a big fan after all. You can find out some really interesting things about your likes and dislikes through this.

For many people, eating this way helps them to feel more satisfied, and reduces the chance of experiencing that sensation of wanting more after a meal, even though they feel physically full. But mindful eating is not a tool for eliminating emotional eating. Again, it's something to work alongside it.

Positive food language

You aren't born with negative thoughts about food; you learned them. And that means you can unlearn them. Usually these thoughts have been with us for a while, sometimes since childhood, and as such they've become automatic habits.

Once you've become aware of the language you're using around food and the impact it can have, you can do something about it. Believing in 'bad' food doesn't help you to feel better about yourself; it just causes guilt and anxiety, and leaves you stuck in a place where you can't enjoy food as much, because these negative thoughts taint the experience.

I think it's important to remember that these negative thoughts and feelings around food can lead us to anxiety and thoughts of how to compensate for having eaten something 'bad'. In addition, using words like 'bad' to describe food can lead us to comfort eat, and while there's nothing inherently wrong with comfort eating, it drives a negative cycle of guilt and shame: Eat 'bad' food → guilt → compensate/restrict → get overly hungry → see bad food → eat → guilt … and so on.

Remember, food is morally neutral; it does not make you a good or bad person. Giving a food the label 'good' doesn't make it morally superior to others, although it certainly creates that illusion. Moralising food takes away the enjoyment of it. It's deciding whether you are or aren't allowed to enjoy something based on a dichotomy and judgement that doesn't exist. Be honest with yourself: if you stop calling that dessert 'bad', how much more are you going to be able to enjoy it and savour it?

Telling yourself there are no good or bad foods is one thing, but the way to consolidate that is by putting it into practice. You have to back up your thoughts with actions. Try it – see how it feels.

So, if thinking of foods as either good or bad doesn't actually help you to eat better, then what does? In my experience, it's eating observantly, but non-judgementally, and taking note of your pleasure both during and after eating. Noticing both how food tastes during eating and how it makes you feel, physically, after. Over time, with experimentation, the black-and-white terms you use to describe food become less prevalent, and the feelings of guilt are replaced with pleasure. This takes time and continuous practice, and you have to keep reminding yourself that food isn't simply good or bad, clean or dirty, real or fake. And you have to believe that it cannot, by association, make you good or bad either.

Changing thoughts is what we have power over, and we can change thoughts through language. It may sound scary, but it starts by counting automatic negative thoughts around food and eating. Recognise these thoughts, then replace them with something positive. I've offered some suggestions below, but if you don't like the words or phrases I've used, feel free to create your own. The point is that you have to believe it.

NEGATIVE WORDS OR PHRASES	POSITIVE WORDS OR PHRASES
Clean	Delicious
'Real' food	Wonderful
Detox/cleanse	Everyday/occasional food
Cheat meal/day	Fun foods
Guilt-free	Balanced
Empty calories	Tasty
Good/bad	More/less nutritious
Healthy/unhealthy	Enjoyable
Naughty	Fun
Junk food	Well-cooked
'Earn your food'	Spicy/crispy/smooth/creamy
Nasties	Satisfying
Fattening	Nourishing
Decadent	Appetising
Sinful	Fresh
My weakness	Exciting
Forbidden/allowed	Yum
Toxic	Comforting
Reward	Filling
Addictive	Pleasurable
I shouldn't	I want to

Making these changes to how you talk about food isn't just beneficial for you and your mental health, it's also beneficial to those around you who hear your comments. The language you use can lead others to feel either guilty or happy about the fact that you're enjoying something delicious. Young people in particular can be positively or negatively influenced by your comments. To any parents reading this: I don't want to scare you, but to issue a gentle reminder that the language you use to talk about yourself and food will be picked up by your children, and will shape their ideas about themselves and eating. Being a positive role model for your children can have huge benefits, and allows them to thrive in a home environment where they are taught that food is wonderful, not something to be afraid of, and that their self-worth comes from more than just their appearance.

Saying 'You shouldn't eat that', for example, if they want ice cream, firstly introduces the idea of guilt and shame around food choices, and secondly makes that food so much more desirable because it's forbidden. Although it's not as obvious as putting your child on a diet, it's encouraging diet mentality of 'good' and 'bad' foods, and a deprivation-overeat mindset.

On a more obvious note, ask yourself whether you speak about weight, dieting and body image in front of your children. Do you say there are certain foods you aren't 'allowed' but then feed these foods to your family? Think of how a child might feel if they're eating something you've said you're trying to avoid. How do you think they may interpret that? It's confusing for them, and although they might not be able to articulate it, these ideas are internalised. It's why in my first session with a new client I'll dedicate time to asking them about their relationship with food while growing up. I'll find out what they can remember about how their parents spoke about food and weight, what they learned from that, and how it affected them. Because it does affect them – hugely in some cases, barely in others, but it's a risk all the same. Using words like 'strong', 'balanced' or 'beautiful' to speak to them and to speak about yourself makes such a difference, as how you speak about these topics becomes the child's new 'normal'.

There are so many moral, loaded terms we use to describe food. Even the word 'carbs' has negative associations for a lot of people. Why don't we just call food what it is? That's not a guilty pleasure, it's a piece of cake. It's not a carb, it's a potato. That's not a healthy option, it's just a goddamn apple. Call a spade a spade. Food is far more than just one moral judgement or one type of nutrient. It's food. Call it by its name.

Orthorexia

Individuals with orthorexia or orthorexic tendencies can really benefit from the tools to reshape the way we think and talk about food. When I typically help people in clinic with ortho-rexic tendencies, the most important factor is addressing food fears and food anxieties. This isn't something that's unique to people with orthorexia, though; when I see chronic dieters in clinic, the same guidance applies. Regardless of whether you have orthorexia or not, thanks to diet culture most of us will have some disordered attitudes towards food, and addressing these will lead to better mental and physical health.

First, you have to be honest with yourself, and find out what foods you feel you can't eat. Or, if that doesn't work for you, write a list of foods that make you feel guilty when you eat them. Next to each one, note what it is about that food that makes you feel guilty or feel like you can't eat it, and where you think that idea came from.

For example:

- Doughnuts – why? Too high in sugar. Where did it come from? Various articles and tweets.
- Pizza – why? Not enough vegetables. Where did it come from? Comments from co-workers.

Second, I think it's important to understand that health is about more than just the nutrients in our food. As I have done in this book, with clients I try to establish an overall picture of what health is, and all the various factors that contribute to it, such as a social life, stress, sleep and so on. This helps place nutrition in context, rather than it being the sole determinant of health in someone's mind. The goal is to reduce the power of food, so that instead of it being the centre of everything, it simply becomes one part of life, one small part of the puzzle; and to develop an understanding and practice of moderation that allows for eating a healthy diet without it becoming addictive and an impossible quest for total perfection.

Finally, I think it's important to understand why someone has developed orthorexia. We are all subject to the same cultural messages prizing health and thinness, yet many of us don't go on to develop eating disorders. This process involves uncovering anxieties, issues with self-esteem and perfectionism, and the many other very human problems that someone with orthorexia will have been attempting to manage through food alone. This is also why I recommend seeing both a nutritionist and a psychologist or therapist, as ideally the two need to work together.

If you think you have orthorexia, some of these tools may help you, but I want to encourage you to seek professional guidance, as it's really challenging to do this on your own. You deserve to feel better, and you deserve to get the best help you can to get you there.

Fearmongering

If you haven't been surrounded by messages that carbohydrates and sugar are deadly poisons, consider yourself lucky. As a nutritionist who tries to stay on top of both the latest research and the latest diet trends, not a day goes by that I don't see some foods or nutrients being demonised and falsely labelled as 'evil', 'disease-causing', 'toxic' or any other fearmongering word.

As I mentioned, a healthy relationship with food doesn't involve guilt, and nor should it involve fear. Fear is not a constructive emotion to feel around food, although it may have been, far back in the history of our evolution. Feeling fear takes away from the enjoyment of food and eating.

If someone is making you feel fear or anxiety about eating something that you have no legitimate medical reason to avoid, they are a negative influence on your life.

Fear is arguably the most effective marketing tool there is. We fear gaining weight and becoming fat because society has told us that's the worst thing a person can be. Equally we fear becoming unwell because then we're a drain on the NHS and are afraid we'll be told it's all our own fault.

- If foods like bread and pasta really are evil, why has Italy managed just fine eating these pretty much daily?
- If rice is such a useless food, so devoid of nutrition, then why do billions of people in Asia and India not suffer as a result of eating lots of it every day?
- If cheese is so dangerous for human consumption, why don't countries such as France, Italy, Spain or Switzerland have much higher rates of diet-related disease?

Demonising individual foods or nutrients is a big problem. It doesn't make people healthier and doesn't promote a healthy relationship with food. In fact, I would argue it makes people less healthy, both mentally and physically.

Obviously, as a nutritionist I'm well aware that there are certain foods we perhaps should be eating less of, and certain others we should be emphasising, all while taking into account the context of an entire diet and other factors that affect health. But this is nuanced, it's not black and white, and it's not as simple as cutting out a food and magically being healthy.

There are two main reasons I think food fearmongering has become so prevalent:

1. Sensationalist fearmongering sells. If you want to make money selling diet books or a TV series, then fear is essential. Many of the extreme fearmongering views that spread are from people who are trying to sell you something, and that is their primary goal: making money. Not your health. It's there

to make you feel bad, because fear drives profits. If you're scared that bread will give you diabetes, you're more likely to read the books and buy the supplements and the meal plans.

2. We like simple messages. Nutrition is complex, and we don't like that. It's far simpler to say more and more people are developing diabetes because of sugar (even though our sugar consumption is actually going down...), or that people are getting cancer because of pesticides (never mind that organic food also uses pesticides...). The concept of moderation is dull; there is no real way of making it sexy, but I try.

It also allows us to play the blame game. Demonising individual foods allows us to praise ourselves for being morally superior and healthier because we're not eating a particular food, and look down on others who do eat it, as we frame it as 'They're making themselves sick.' I've lost count of how many hateful comments I've seen along the lines of 'She eats meat – no wonder she got cancer' or 'If only she'd started juicing, this wouldn't have happened,' as if the only reason you don't get cancer is because of the way you eat. No mention of genetics or social determinants or anything.

That same blame game is what drives the stereotype of fat people as being lazy and unmotivated, because it's their fault they got fat. It also drives the narrative of fat people being a burden on the NHS, because it makes us feel better about our bodies and our choices. It doesn't matter that it isn't true, because it's a defence mechanism that makes us feel better, so we don't question it.

All this fearmongering creates food phobias and drives fat-phobia. It makes people afraid of eating fruit because of sugar, or afraid to eat bread because of carbs, or beans because of lectins. These fearmongering messages cause real psychological harm, and then it's up to people like me to do the hard work of trying to reassure someone that it's ok for them to eat this food – it won't hurt them. Inducing fear of food takes a second, but undoing that can take months or years. Not only that, but it hurts people physically as well, as it makes them stressed and can lead to deficiencies as a result of cutting out foods. Fearmongering causes real harm.

Fearmongering creates confusion. Every charlatan, every diet book, every 'guru' has a different set of rules to follow and a different food to be afraid of. No wonder people are confused. If you followed all their advice at the same time, there wouldn't be a single food left you could eat (oh I checked). I see countless people in clinic who have followed every diet they could think of and now they have the most confusing conflicting rules in their head, and it drives them to despair. And I get questions daily on social media along the lines of 'Is it ok for me to eat this?' It really makes me sad, and it makes me really angry.

If you feel as angry as I do about this, then speak up and say something when you see this kind of fearmongering happening. Make it clear you are against overly simplistic, fearful, out-of-context dietary messages and vocalise your thoughts about how damaging they are. Food isn't toxic, but what is toxic is spreading fear-inducing, one-dimensional dietary messages in the name of profit.

How to protect yourself against fearmongering tactics

Unfortunately, there's no simple solution to recognising and avoiding fearmongering, but there are some things that can help. First, recognise that you are human, and that we all fall for bullshit sometimes. None of us is infallible, but what we can do is commit to being more sceptical and questioning of what we read. Don't take something at face value just because it sounds plausible. Particularly, question what you read online. Does someone have the qualifications to back up what they're saying? Where is the research? Does it sound too good to be true?

I think it's easy to suffer from nutrition information overload, and a lot of us could do with reading a little bit less about nutrition. If you see a sensationalist headline, try to ignore it – don't immediately feel the need to read it. The same goes for social media. And most of all, don't get your nutrition information from Netflix.

If you follow someone or see something that's using fear to get you to change, recognise it, ignore it or unfollow it, and move on.

Social media

The only time the word 'detox' is acceptable is when it's prefaced by the words 'social media'. I cannot recommend social media detoxes enough.

It's important to recognise all the negatives of social media: the social comparison, the risk of depression and eating disorders, and the obsessive nature it encourages. But there is also the good, and if you can shape your social-media experience you can tip the scales in the right direction.

We know that spending too much time on social media isn't

good for our mental health, so if you find you're spending more than an hour per day on a single social-media platform, I'd recommend cutting down. If you're unaware of how much time you spend on social media, I have a tip for iPhone users. On your settings, go to 'battery' and gasp in horror, as it tells you your total screen time, as well as how much time you've spent on each app in the last twenty-four hours and in the last seven days.

The first time I checked this I was horrified at how many hours (yes, hours) I was spending on Twitter and Instagram. It's eye-opening. Since then I've really tried hard to spend less time on those apps, even though, to some extent, my work depends on it.

Here are some quick tips I often use and recommend to reduce the time I spend on social media:

- On public transport, put a podcast or music on and switch to Flight Mode.
- Walk with your phone in your bag and don't take it out (unless you're lost).
- Put your phone on Flight Mode at the gym or when going for a run.
- When eating at home, leave your phone in another room, even if you're alone.
- When eating out, leave your phone in your bag. Don't even let it sit on the table.
- Turn off all push notifications apart from texts/messages from important people.

I know these sound super simple and straightforward, but sometimes we need someone to tell us these things, and need them spelled out in black and white in order for us to make a change. Social media is a habit for most of us, and habits are hard to break.

If you feel more extreme action is needed, then consider apps that block you out of your social media apps after a certain time, which you decide on beforehand. Or there are apps such as 'Forest', which will plant a tree if you ignore your phone for a consecutive two-hour period. How incredible is that?

As an experiment, delete your social media apps for twenty-four hours and see how you feel. Or next time you go away for a weekend, delete them for the whole time. I can guarantee you'll feel refreshed, happier, and like you have so much more time in the day.

Right now, I can perfectly picture most of you thinking 'Sure I'm on social media, but I'm not addicted to my phone – I'm not obsessed'. In that case, I offer you a challenge. If you have an iPhone, you can now track your usage and even track how many notifications you get daily. Or you can download an app like Moment (iOS) or MyAddictometer (Android) and track your usage for a few days. It'll even send out handy notifications so you don't forget about it. Do the results surprise you? If they do, it means you're using your phone and using social media far more than you thought, and could save yourself a lot of time by being more mindful of it. Not only that, but the less time you're spending on social media, the fewer opportunities there are for upward social comparison, FOMO, and worse mood.

Taking a break from social media frees up time and mental space you weren't even aware you had lost. Doing a social media detox puts you back in control of how you use these platforms, and enables you to use them more positively and mindfully.

Aside from how much time you spend on social media, it's also important to assess the kind of content you consume. Is every person you follow on social media a thin white person? If yes, it's time to add some diversity. Make your feed represent the real world with all its variation: fat people, minority ethnic groups, LGBTQ+ folks, trans folks, disabled folks... Let your social media feed remind you of how wonderfully different we all are.

Do you follow people who make you feel bad about yourself? Unfollow these people. For every one of them you remove, replace it with plants or fluffy animals or nature or art.

Does everyone you follow eat the same way as you? That's not realistic. No matter if you're vegan or paleo, the whole world doesn't eat the way you do, and only following people who do what you do creates an echo chamber that never allows you to be challenged in any way.

Media

Exposure to ideal body shapes in the media is a definite risk factor for mental health issues like low self-esteem, poor body image, depression and eating disorders. Based on that, reducing or eliminating (as much as possible) these negative media influences should help negate some of this risk. One method is simply to drastically reduce the amount of media you consume. Stop buying magazines, especially ones that claim to be about health while promoting nothing but weight loss and muscle gain – there's nothing healthy about these. Don't watch TV with adverts – either use the ad time to get up and do something else, or record the show and fast-forward. And stop reading news articles about nutrition in general; nine times out of ten they're unhelpful and wrong anyway.

Another method that's been proposed, which may help counter some of the negative effects of the media, is media literacy training. Media literacy is a set of knowledge, attitudes and skills that enables someone to understand, appreciate and critically analyse the nature of mass media and their relationships with these media. More specifically, it helps with several ideas:

- Learning to think critically and be sceptical about the information you see. This involves deciding whether the messages make sense, why certain information was included, whether anything was left out, and what the key ideas are.

- Becoming a smart consumer of products and information. Media literacy helps people learn how to determine whether something is credible, and potentially resist the techniques used in advertising.

- Creating media responsibly. Not just passively consuming, but also recognising what you want to say and how you want that information to be conveyed.

- Identifying the role of media in our culture. From celebrity gossip to magazine covers to memes, media is telling us something, shaping our understanding of the world, and even compelling us to act or think in certain ways.

- Understanding the author's goal. What does the author want you to take away from a piece of media? Is it purely informative? Is it trying to change your mind about something? The media helps shape our understanding of the world, and understanding people's intentions is key.

Several experiments show that media literacy training can protect women against feeling worse about themselves after viewing ideal bodies in the media, even if they already have negative body image. The most effective methods highlight the differences between the artificial, constructed nature of the ideal body compared with the natural diversity of human body shapes, and compared with the actual reality of diets and the negative effects of them. Media literacy programmes that span the course of a month or two in schools can help reduce the risk of internalising the thin or lean ideal, as well as increase self-acceptance and self-confidence.[112]

Several researchers have developed a four-week media literacy course, which involves discussing how beauty ideals are presented in the media, learning about the nature and causes of body dissatisfaction, awareness of photo editing and beauty enhancement, and a brief cognitive intervention designed to help dispute negative beliefs and feelings that come from media images of ideal bodies. This has proved to be highly successful in reducing risk factors for disordered eating, such as unhealthy social attitudes, internalisation of the thin or lean ideal and body dissatisfaction.

What we ideally need is media literacy training to be compulsory in schools. That in itself would make a huge difference. However it doesn't help you at the present time. Here's what you can do right now. As adults, we can still use the principles of media literacy to ask three important questions when we read something in the media: Who's the author? What's the purpose of this message? How was this message constructed?

I also think it's important for us to read articles that we don't agree with. It may feel infuriating but it's important that we understand others' points of view and listen. Even if we think someone is spouting total bollocks, it's still useful to know these viewpoints exist and how prevalent they are. This is also why I've mentioned that it's important to follow people on social media who eat and think differently from you – it gets you out of an echo chamber where your beliefs are simply being reinforced without question, and where you may be led to believe your views are more prevalent than they actually are.

We find it very difficult to read things that we disagree with. Our natural inclination is to seek out things we agree with, also known as confirmation bias. If something agrees with you it's wonderful and correct; if it disagrees with you it must be flawed or biased in some way. Overcoming that bias is hard, but it's the mark of a good sceptic. Whatever beliefs you hold, particularly around food and health, particularly ones you hold tightly, you should take the time to actively try to prove them wrong. Actively seek out research that disagrees with you. Sounds scary, but the outcome is either that you can't find compelling evidence to say you're wrong, in which case keep going with your viewpoint; or you find plenty of evidence that proves you wrong, in which case you can modify your standpoint to reflect the totality of the evidence. Either way, you end up with a viewpoint that is backed by evidence and that you can be even more sure of as a result. It's a win-win situation, but it's far easier said than done.

I don't think it's realistic to expect people to never consume any media messages ever. It's impossible – you might walk in on your flatmate or family member watching something on TV, videos get shared on social media, billboards are all over the place, and besides, it's fun to watch TV! Not all popular media is problematic – obviously, I couldn't possibly have a bad word to say about anything by David Attenborough, for example. Perhaps what we need is greater awareness of what we watch, and to take some time to assess whether what we are watching shows enough diversity in humans and in bodies.

Healthy movement

Moving your body is a wonderful thing, and carries with it a whole host of benefits, both mental and physical. Focusing on these health benefits rather than aesthetics as your primary motivation for exercise means you'll have better body image and overall mental health.

This also means moving away from the idea of exercise as punishment. That attitude doesn't work for most of us – just think back to PE classes. Sports teachers often use punishments such as doing extra laps, but this just creates a negative association with exercise. It doesn't motivate and encourage more movement, and neither does fitspo. Fitspo teaches us that our fitness goals should be focused on how we look, and that there is only one way to have a fit body.

None of this encourages a healthy attitude towards exercise. Here is what does: moving in a way that feels good for your body. Not based on what some fitness tracker says, not doing what fitspos are doing, not what Google says will burn the most calories in one hour. Simply what you enjoy and what feels good in your body, which is different for everyone. It can even vary within the same person from year to year. To use myself as an example, I went through a period of loving spin and boot-camp classes, then when that became too expensive I switched to weights sessions at the gym. After a time, though, I realised these sessions were just making me feel tired and even more stressed, and too focused on increasing my weights, which left me disheartened when my progress stalled. So I switched to yoga, which has done wonders for my stress levels and overall mental health. That's where I'm at now, but it might change again next year, and that's totally ok. I'm listening to my body, and it makes me happier. Pleasure is a much more powerful long-term motivator than guilt and pain.

Some people find focusing on functionality incredibly moti-vating when it comes to exercise. I once heard a personal trainer say, 'We do squats so that when we're eighty years old we can still get up off the toilet by ourselves', and that really stuck with me. The focus wasn't on having a peachy bum – it was on being independent for as long as possible. For others, though, this focus isn't helpful; it's actually quite ableist. Many disabled folks are all too aware of what their body can't do, and how well it doesn't function, so focusing on that can actually be detrimental. This is why thinking about the mental health benefits of simply being outside in nature, or doing a short walk or a gentle stretch, are also worth stressing.

For those of you who are able, think about how it feels when you move your body. Does it feel good? Does it feel too easy or too hard? Does it leave you feeling tired but happy? Or does it make you unproductive for the rest of the day? Does it help with stress or make it worse? Do you enjoy moving more in the morning or afternoon? Are you having fun? Are you taking enough time to rest as well as move?

Rest is so important. Rest is physically essential for your muscles to repair, rebuild and strengthen. When you exercise, you break down muscle tissue and cause micro-tears in muscle tissue, which need time to repair. You also deplete your glycogen stores – the carbohydrate-based energy stores in your muscles – and lose fluids, which need time to replenish. Without enough time to do this, the body will continue to break down instead of repair. It's essential to listen to your body and gauge how you're feeling. If you're tired, then rest. Otherwise you might even end up injuring yourself.

Finally, I want to make a point about uncoupling exercise from weight loss. Not only is exercise by itself a really slow and disheartening method for weight loss, we already know that focusing on weight loss doesn't work. We need to stop conflating the two, and assuming that everyone who exercises does it for weight loss or weight maintenance. It's kind of insulting to us as complex humans.

Body image

Social media, the media and fitspo can all contribute to negative body image through social comparison. I've talked about body image in the context of these platforms, but it deserves to be talked about in its own right.

There has been a huge 'body positivity' movement in recent years, but it's been twisted and distorted from its original purpose. Many people incorrectly believe that body positivity is simply about loving your body, but it's so much more than that. It's a political movement founded by fat black women with the intention of celebrating marginalised bodies who aren't commonly seen in mainstream media. It was started to create a safe space for non-privileged bodies to be celebrated, as no such place existed otherwise. This is the key difference: the body positivity movement was created for marginalised bodies; positive body image and appreciating the body you're in is for everyone. Some say the movement should have been called 'fat acceptance' instead, as that way it wouldn't have been appropriated by others. I'm inclined to agree.

Negative body image doesn't discriminate on grounds of shape or size. Everyone can be negatively affected by body dissatisfaction and even body hatred. Nobody is suggesting that thin people can't have problems with their bodies and self-esteem; the key difference is that their bodies are accepted and even praised by society (as a general rule), whereas fat bodies are not.

I hope that makes things clearer. Now, on to body image itself. Positive body image does not necessarily mean loving yourself. For many people, that is an unrealistic goal, especially short term. If you were to look at yourself in the mirror right now and say 'I love myself', would you believe it? If yes, go you! Keep hold of that. If not, that's ok, you don't have to love yourself. Instead, what I find a more realistic goal is body acceptance, or body neutrality.

Body neutrality is about simply accepting yourself the way you are. It means feeling pretty neutral towards it – neither loving it nor disliking it, but rather not really thinking about it that much because it's just there and you move on with your day. Having body acceptance and good body image means taking the time to do nice things for your body, but not obsessing over it. It's treating your body with respect because you believe (or are trying to believe) that it deserves to be treated well. In practice, this can mean countering negative thoughts about your body (more on that in a bit), wearing clothes that fit well and feel comfortable, feeding your body when it's hungry, resting it when it needs to rest, and not poking and prodding at bits you don't like.

A lot of us have automatic negative thoughts about our bodies. We look in the mirror and are immediately drawn to parts we don't like or that we feel aren't good enough. With my clients, I like to do an exercise where I get them to make a tally (either in writing or on their phone) every time they think something negative about their body. At the end of the day, they add them all up and are usually shocked by just how often they have these thoughts. The next step after that is to try to counter each negative thought with a positive or neutral one. For example, replace 'I hate my thighs' with 'These thighs carried me to work and back today'. Not overwhelmingly positive and exciting, but accurate, and showing appreciation.

Our perception becomes our reality. If we can change our perceptions about our body and see it in a neutral or positive light, that then becomes our reality and we feel more comfortable in the body we have. It's not an overnight process – it takes time – but it's so worth it.

There are several ways we can work at improving our body image. Countering negative thoughts is one. Moving our bodies in a way that we enjoy, without focusing on aesthetics, is another. We can also do nice things for ourselves in the form of self-care, as I mentioned above in the section on emotional eating (see 'Satisfy your needs', page 251). And there's also self-compassion.

Self-compassion expert Dr Kristin Neff has defined self-compassion as being composed of three main components: self-kindness, common humanity and mindfulness.

Self-kindness means being warm and kind towards yourself even when you're experiencing pain, you've done something wrong, or you've failed. Instead of criticising yourself for not being good enough, it's about comforting yourself and telling yourself it's ok. Think of it as treating yourself how you would a friend.

Common humanity means recognising that suffering and failure is part of the shared human experience. To be human means to be imperfect, and that is shared among all humans. Reminding ourselves of that can help us feel less like an outcast, because failure is normal. There's something so relieving about hearing someone say, 'I feel that too.' It makes us feel less alone.

Mindfulness means observing that, yes, there is pain and you are suffering, and simply seeing that in a non-judgemental light. Thoughts and feelings, especially negative ones, are not denied but accepted. We get so lost in our own self-criticism that we often don't notice the negative effects that has. Mindfulness doesn't mean sulking or ruminating over what you've said and done, but simply accepting and moving on to kinder thoughts.

How can you put this into practice? One of the best ways is to imagine a friend is in your situation. As an example, let's say you failed an exam. Your negative self-talk might be saying: 'You're a failure. This is awful. How could you let this happen?' But would you say that to a friend? I very much doubt it. Instead, you might say to that friend: 'I understand this is horrible for you – I've been there too. You'll have another chance to resit this exam. Do you want me to help you study?' Based on that, to yourself you might then choose to say: 'Yes, this isn't what I wanted, and it hurts and it's a horrible situation, but it's not the end of the world. People fail all the time. I know I have another shot at this exam, and I'm going to study harder because I know I can do better.' This is realistic; it's not making the situation out to be anything it isn't, and it's so much kinder.

We often believe that being self-critical and harsh to ourselves is motivating, but in fact it does the opposite. Self-criticism makes us both the attacker and the attacked. That makes us stressed and less able to function. Telling yourself you're a failure is more likely to make you depressed and feel helpless than it is to get you motivated. But being kind to yourself is giving yourself hope and having faith in yourself. And the research shows it's far more effective in the long run.

It makes sense that self-compassion would help mitigate some of the suffering associated with body dissatisfaction, as it's a strategy that encourages people to accept themselves regardless of any imperfections, regardless of their achievements and regardless of their failures. The self-critical voice associated with body dissatisfaction tells you that your body isn't good enough, whereas self-compassion and self-kindness say it is. Similarly, the common humanity in knowing that almost everyone feels this way about their body at some point in their lives can be reassuring that you're not weird. The mindfulness aspect then helps to assess these thoughts in a balanced, non-judgemental way rather than fixating over body parts that are disliked. So self-compassion can actually fight body dissatisfaction and help people to appreciate and accept their bodies with all the perceived flaws.[177] It can also help improve body image by offering women in particular another way of valuing themselves that doesn't involve their physical appearance, as self-compassion is associated with greater optimism and life satisfaction.[178]

Women's self-esteem, and men's to a growing extent, is quite heavily dependent on meeting societal standards of ideal beauty. If these standards aren't met, then we might be called ugly or fat (in a derogatory sense rather than as a neutral descriptor), and our self-worth can suffer as a result. In this instance, while self-esteem would be knocked due to failing to meet a particular standard, self-compassion can help, as it involves treating ourselves kindly, especially in times of adversity when self-esteem is lowered. Self-compassion is not dependent on coming out well in social comparisons; it is less affected by it and can actually help prevent it. Women who practise self-compassion are less likely to worry about their bodies or their weight; in fact, they're more likely to appreciate their bodies, even when they evaluate their bodies as inferior to another. They're also less judgemental when they have low self-esteem.[179]

Overall, self-compassion has a great many upsides, without any of the pitfalls that come with self-esteem, as self-compassion isn't dependent on any success or accomplishments, and helps you thrive despite failings and perceived shortcomings.

The final point I want to share on fostering positive body image is that it can be incredibly helpful to surround yourself with people trying to achieve the same goal. Create a healthy distance between yourself and people focused on changing their bodies, wherever possible, and find a community either online or offline who are doing what you're doing. Follow some amazing people online who are loving their bodies, or join a Facebook group for support. It can be so motivating to see other people around you who aren't just losing weight and moulding their bodies but are accepting and embracing them instead.

The bigger picture

Nutrition is important. As a nutritionist, I obviously believe that and have dedicated a great deal of time to studying and understanding it. But then I see quotes like 'Every bite you take is either fighting disease or feeding it,' usually with a picture of a vegetable and a burger getting into a fight. These kinds of quotes, and any other 'food is medicine' rhetoric, are incredibly oversimplifying something as complex as health. There is so much more to health than just the food you eat. There are factors like sleep and stress, which have huge effects on our appetite and food choices. Then there are the independent links between stress and disease, and sleep and disease, which don't involve food at all. Not to mention the importance of social health, happiness, medical care, genetics and socio-economic factors, all of which are largely out of our hands. You could spend all your life making sure you had the most optimised diet, exercise pattern and sleep schedule possible, but you won't be immortal. In fact, you'll probably live to a hundred and be miserable because you have no friends, and then die of cancer anyway. Or you'll die of a heart attack at forty because of all the stress and worry. Where is the fun in that? What is the point of life if it's not to be lived and enjoyed. I don't believe in gods or some higher power; I don't believe in there being some great purpose for us all being here. I think we're all just here because of the laws of physics and probability, but that doesn't mean we can't have fun while it lasts. And food is fun. Oh, so much fun.

You were not put on this earth to devote all your energy into looking a certain way. Think of all the amazing things you could do if you spent less time worrying about food. You don't have to change the world or do something to put you into the history books. Just do things that make your life exciting and worthwhile, so that when you get to the end of it you don't feel like you've wasted your chance at life.

When you die, no one is going to remember you for your crazy gym routine, or for what you ate, or for your weight. People will remember you for the kind things you did for them.

Yes, your health is important, but health isn't a moral imperative or an obligation. Human beings are deserving of basic respect, regardless of whether they are healthy or not. People with genetic disorders or chronic illnesses may not fit the bill of 'health' but they are still humans. Someone in a larger body deserves equal kindness and respect. These things are unconditional, not dependent on health status.

Society tells us the worst thing you can be is fat. They are wrong. The worst thing you can be is inconsiderate and judgemental and unkind to others.

BIBLIOGRAPHY

1. Flegal, K.M., Kit, B.K., Orpana, H., Graubard, B.I. (2013). 'Association of all-cause mortality with overweight and obesity using standard body mass index categories'. *JAMA*, 309(1):71.
2. Bacon, L., Aphramor, L. (2011). 'Weight science: Evaluating the evidence for a paradigm shift'. *Nutrition Journal*, 10(1):9.
3. Wing, R.R., Phelan, S. 'Long-term weight loss maintenance'. (2005). *The American Journal of Clinical Nutrition*, 82(1):222S–225S.
4. Howard, B. V., Manson, J.E., Stefanick, M.L, et al. (2006). 'Low-fat dietary pattern and weight change over seven years'. *JAMA*, 295(1):39.
5. NIH Technology Assessment Conference Panel. (1992). 'Methods for voluntary weight loss and control'. *Annals of Internal Medicine*, 116(11):942–949.
6. Mann, T., Tomiyama, A.J., Westling, E., Lew, A-M, Samuels, B., Chatman, J. (2007). 'Medicare's search for effective obesity treatments: Diets are not the answer'. *American Psychologist*, 62(3): 220–233.
7. French, S.A., Jeffery, R.W., Forster, J.L. (1994). 'Dieting status and its relationship to weight, dietary intake, and physical activity changes over two years in a working population'. *Obesity Research & Clinical Practice*, 2(2):135–144.
8. Fisher, J.O., Birch, L.L. (1999). Restricting access to palatable foods affects children's behavioral response, food selection, and intake'. *The American Journal of Clinical Nutrition*, (6):1264–1272.
9. Tsai, A.G., Wadden, T.A. (2005). 'Systematic review: An evaluation of major commercial weight loss programs in the United States'. *Annals of Internal Medicine*, 142(1):56.

10. James, J., Thomas, P., Kerr, D. (2007). 'Preventing childhood obesity: Two year follow-up results from the Christchurch obesity prevention programme in schools (CHOPPS)'. *BMJ*, 335(7623):762.

11. Anderson, L.M., Quinn, T.A., Glanz K., et al. (2009). 'The effectiveness of worksite nutrition and physical activity interventions for controlling employee overweight and obesity'. *American Journal of Preventative Medicine*, 37(4):340–357.

12. Bosomworth, N.J. (2012). 'The downside of weight loss: Realistic intervention in body-weight trajectory'. *Canadian Family Physician*, 58(5):517–523.

13. Aphramor, L. (2010). 'Validity of claims made in weight management research: A narrative review of dietetic articles'. *Nutrition Journal*, 9:30. doi:10.1186/1475-2891-9-30.

14. Müller, M.J., Bosy-Westphal, A., Heymsfield, S.B. (2010). 'Is there evidence for a set point that regulates human body weight?' *F1000 Medicine Reports*, 2:59.

15. Polivy, J., Herman, C.P. (1985). 'Dieting and binging: A causal analysis'. *American Psychologist*, 40(2):193–201.

16. Leibel, R.L., Hirsch, J. (1984). 'Diminished energy requirements in reduced-obese patients'. *Metabolism*, 33(2):164–170.

17. Sumithran, P., Prendergast, L.A., Delbridge, E., et al. (2011). 'Long-term persistence of hormonal adaptations to Weight Loss'. *The New England Journal of Medicine*, 365(17):1597–1604.

18. Bacon, L., Stern, J.S., Van Loan, M.D., Keim, N.L. (2005). 'Size acceptance and intuitive eating improve health for obese, female chronic dieters'. *Journal of the American Dietetic Association*, 105(6): 929–936.

19. Khaw, K-T, Wareham, N., Bingham, S., Welch, A., Luben, R., Day, N. (2008). 'Combined impact of health behaviours and mortality in men and women: The EPIC-Norfolk prospective population study'. Lopez A, ed. *PLoS Medicine*, 5(1):e12.

20. Matheson, E.M., King, D.E., Everett, C.J. (2012). 'Healthy lifestyle habits and mortality in overweight and obese individuals'. *Journal of the American Board of Family Medicine*, 25(1):9–15.

21. Rothblum, E.D. (2018). 'Slim chance for permanent weight loss'. *Archives of Scientific Psychology*, 6(1):63–69.

22. Fox, R. (2018). 'Against progress: Understanding and resisting

the temporality of transformational weight loss narratives'. *Fat Studies*, 7(2):216–226.

23.   Lissner, L., Odell, P.M., D'Agostino, R.B., et al. (1991). 'Variability of Body Weight and Health Outcomes in the Framingham Population'. *The New England Journal of Medicine*, 324(26):1839–1844.

24.   Brownell, K.D., Rodin, J. (1994). 'Medical, metabolic, and psychological effects of weight cycling'. *Archives of Internal Medicine*, 154(12):1325–1330.

25.   Field, A.E., Manson, J.E., Taylor, C.B., Willett, W.C., Colditz, G.A. (2004). 'Association of weight change, weight control practices and weight cycling among women in the Nurses' Health Study II. *International Journal of Obesity*, 28(9):1134–1142.

26.   Andreyeva, T., Puhl, R.M., Brownell, K.D. (2008). 'Changes in perceived weight discrimination among Americans, 1995–1996 through 2004–2006'. *Obesity*, 16(5):1129–1134.

27.   Davis-Coelho, K., Waltz, J., Davis-Coelho, B. (2000). 'Awareness and prevention of bias against fat clients in psychotherapy'. *Professional Psychology Research and Practice*, 31(6):682–684.

28.   Swift, J.A., Hanlon, S., El-Redy, L., Puhl, R.M., Glazebrook, C. (2013). 'Weight bias among UK trainee dietitians, doctors, nurses and nutritionists'. *Journal of Human Nutrition and Dietetics*, 26(4): 395–402.

29.   Stice, E., Presnell, K., Spangler, D. (2002). 'Risk factors for binge eating onset in adolescent girls: a 2-year prospective investigation'. *Health Psychology*, 21(2):131–138.

30.   Tylka, TL. (2011). 'Refinement of the tripartite influence model for men: Dual body image pathways to body change behaviors'. *Body Image*, 8(3):199–207.

31.   Pearl, R.L., Wadden, T.A., Hopkins, C.M., et al. (2017). 'Association between weight bias internalization and metabolic syndrome among treatment-seeking individuals with obesity'. *Obesity*, 25(2):317–322.

32.   Mottillo, S., Filion, K.B., Genest, J., et al. (2010). 'The metabolic syndrome and cardiovascular risk'. *Journal of the American College of Cardiology*, 56(14):1113–1132.

33.   Sutin, A.R., Stephan, Y., Terracciano, A. (2015). 'Weight discrimination and risk of mortality'. *Psychological Science*, 26(11):1803–1811. doi:10.1177/0956797615601103

34. Puhl, R., Suh, Y. (2015). 'Stigma and eating and weight disorders'. *Current Psychiatry Reports*, 17(3):10.

35. Neumark-Sztainer, D., Bauer, K.W., Friend, S., Hannan, P.J., Story, M., Berge, J.M. (2010). 'Family weight talk and dieting: How much do they matter for body dissatisfaction and disordered eating behaviors in adolescent girls?' *Journal of Adolescent Health*, 47(3):270–276.

36. Vartanian, L.R., Porter, A.M. (2016). 'Weight stigma and eating behavior: A review of the literature'. *Appetite*, 102:3–14.

37. Tylka, T.L., Annunziato, R.A., Burgard, D., et al. (2014). 'The weight-inclusive versus weight-normative approach to health: Evaluating the evidence for prioritizing well-being over weight loss. *Journal of Obesity*.

38. Ramos Salas, X. (2015). 'The ineffectiveness and unintended consequences of the public health war on obesity'. *Canadian Journal of Public Health*, 106(2):e79–81.

39. Lozano-Sufrategui, L., Sparkes, A.C., McKenna, J. (2016). Weighty: NICE's not-so-nice words. *Frontiers in Psychology*, 7:1919.

40. Puhl, R., Peterson, J.L., Luedicke, J. (2013). 'Fighting obesity or obese persons? Public perceptions of obesity-related health messages'. *International Journal of Obesity*, 37(6):774–782.

41. Fikkan, J.L., Rothblum, E.D. (2012). 'Is fat a feminist issue? Exploring the gendered nature of weight bias'. *Sex Roles*, 66(9–10): 575–592.

42. Taheri, S., Lin, L., Austin, D., Young, T., Mignot, E. (2004). 'Short sleep duration is associated with reduced leptin, elevated ghrelin, and increased body mass index'. *PLoS Medicine*, 1(3):e62.

43. Tylka, T.L., Calogero, R.M., Daníelsdóttir, S. (2015). 'Is intuitive eating the same as flexible dietary control? Their links to each other and well-being could provide an answer'. *Appetite*, 95, 166–175.

44. Helliwell, J.F., Layard, R., Sachs, J. (2012). *World Happiness Report*.

45. Vitaliano, P.P., Scanlan, J.M., Zhang, J., Savage, M.V., Hirsch, I.B., Siegler, I.C. (2002). 'A path model of chronic stress, the metabolic syndrome, and coronary heart disease'. *Psychosomatic Medicine*, 64(3):418–435.

46. Oliver, G., Wardle, J. (1999). 'Perceived effects of stress on food choice'. *Physiology & Behavior*, 66(3):511–515.

47. Adam, T.C., Epel, E.S. (2007). 'Stress, eating and the reward system'. *Physiology & Behavior*, 91(4):449–458.

48. Zellner, D.A., Loaiza, S., Gonzalez, Z., et al. (2006). 'Food selection changes under stress'. *Physiology & Behavior*, 87(4):789–793.

49. Kaur, S., Van, A. (2017). 'Do the types of food you eat influence your happiness?' *J UC Merced Undergraduate Research Journal*, 9(2).

50. Tomiyama, A.J., Dallman, M.F., Epel, E.S. (2011). 'Comfort food is comforting to those most stressed: Evidence of the chronic stress response network in high stress women'. *Psychoneuroendocrinology*, 36(10):1513–1519.

51. Troisi, J.D., Gabriel, S. (2011). 'Chicken soup really is good for the soul. *Psychological Science*, 22(6):747–753.

52. Locher, J.L., Yoels, W.C., Maurer, D., van Ells, J. (2005). 'Comfort foods: An exploratory journey into the social and emotional significance of food'. *Food and Foodways*, 13(4):273–297.

53. Spence, C. (2017). 'Comfort food: A review'. *International Journal of Gastronomy and Food Science*, 9:105–109.

54. Macht, M. (1999). 'Characteristics of eating in anger, fear, sadness and joy'. *Appetite*, 33(1):129–139.

55. Macht, M. (2008). 'How emotions affect eating: A five-way model'. *Appetite*, 50(1):1–11.

56. MacCormack, J.K., Lindquist, K.A. (2018). 'Feeling hangry? When hunger is conceptualized as emotion'. *Emotion*. June.

57. Koball, A.M., Meers, M.R., Storfer-Isser, A., Domoff, S.E., Musher-Eizenman, D.R. (2012). 'Eating when bored: Revision of the emotional eating scale with a focus on boredom'. *Journal of Health Psychology*, 31(4):521–524.

58. Havermans, R.C., Vancleef, L., Kalamatianos, A., Nederkoorn, C. (2015). 'Eating and inflicting pain out of boredom'. *Appetite*, 85:52–57.

59. Cardi, V., Leppanen, J., Treasure, J. (2015). 'The effects of negative and positive mood induction on eating behaviour: A meta-analysis of laboratory studies in the healthy population and eating and weight disorders'. *Neuroscience & Biobehavioral Review*, 57:299–309.

60. White, B.A., Horwath, C.C, Conner, T.S. (2013). 'Many apples a day keep the blues away:Daily experiences of negative and positive

affect and food consumption in young adults'. *British Journal of Health Psychology*, 18(4):782–798.

61.　Sánchez-Villegas, A., Henríquez-Sánchez, P., Ruiz-Canela, M., et al. (2015). 'A longitudinal analysis of diet quality scores and the risk of incident depression in the SUN Project'. *BMC Medicine*, 13(1):197.

62.　Jacka, F.N., O'Neil, A., Opie, R., et al. (2017). 'A randomised controlled trial of dietary improvement for adults with major depression (the 'SMILES' trial)'. *BMC Medicine*, 15(1):23.

63.　Wilk, R. (2004). 'Morals and metaphors: the meaning of consumption'. *Elusive Consumption*, 11–26.

64.　Spencer, D.C. (2014). "Eating clean' for a violent body: Mixed martial arts, diet and masculinities'. *Womens Studies International Forum*, 44:247–254.

65.　Zhong, C-B, Liljenquist, K. (2006). 'Washing away your sins: threatened morality and physical cleansing'. *Science*, 313(5792):1451–1452.

66.　Pila, E., Mond, J.M., Griffiths, S., Mitchison, D., Murray, S.B. (2017). 'A thematic content analysis of #cheatmeal images on social media: Characterizing an emerging dietary trend'. *International Journal of Eating Disorders*, 50(6):698–706.

67.　Kuijer, R.G., Boyce, J.A. (2014). 'Chocolate cake. Guilt or celebration? Associations with healthy eating attitudes, perceived behavioural control, intentions and weight-loss'. *Appetite*, 74:48–54.

68.　Varga, M., Thege, B.K., Dukay-Szabó, S., Túry, F., van Furth, E.F. (2014). 'When eating healthy is not healthy: Orthorexia nervosa and its measurement with the ORTO-15 in Hungary'. *BMC Psychiatry*, 14(1).

69.　Dunn, T.M., Bratman, S. (2016). 'On orthorexia nervosa: A review of the literature and proposed diagnostic criteria'. *Eating Behaviors*, 21:11–17.

70.　Moroze, R.M., Dunn, T.M., Craig, Holland, J., Yager, J., Weintraub, P. (2015). 'Microthinking about micronutrients: A case of transition from obsessions about healthy eating to near-fatal "orthorexia nervosa" and proposed diagnostic criteria'. *Psychosomatics*, 56(4): 397–403.

71.　Segura-Garcia, C., Ramacciotti, C., Rania, M., et al. (2015). 'The prevalence of orthorexia nervosa among eating disorder patients after treatment'. *Eating and Weight Disorders*, 20(2):161–166.

72. Barthels F, Meyer F, Huber T, Pietrowsky R. (2017). 'Orthorexic eating behaviour as a coping strategy in patients with anorexia nervosa'. *Eating and Weight Disorders - Studies on Anorexia, Bulimia and Obesity*, 22(2):269-276.

73. Dunn, T.M., Gibbs, J, Whitney, N., Starosta, A. (2017). 'Prevalence of orthorexia nervosa is less than 1%: data from a US sample'. *Eating and Weight Disorders - Studies on Anorexia, Bulimia and Obesity*, 22(1):185-192.

74. Syurina, E.V., Bood, Z.M., Ryman, F.V.M., Muftugil-Yalcin, S. (2018). 'Cultural phenomena believed to be associated with orthorexia nervosa: Opinion study in Dutch health professionals'. *Frontiers in Psychology*, 9:1419.

75. Brytek-Matera, A., Donini, L.M., Krupa, M., Poggiogalle, E., Hay, P. (2015). 'Orthorexia nervosa and self-attitudinal aspects of body image in female and male university students'. *Journal of Eating Disorders*, 3:2.

76. Turner, G., Lefevre, C.E. (2017). 'Instagram use is linked to increased symptoms of orthorexia nervosa'. *Eating and Weight Disorders*.

77. Westwater, M.L., Fletcher, P.C., Ziauddeen, H. (2016). 'Sugar addiction: the state of the science'. *European Journal of Nutrition*, 55(S2): 55-69.

78. Biesiekierski, J.R., Peters, S.L., Newnham, E.D., Rosella, O., Muir, J.G., Gibson, P.R. (2013). 'No effects of gluten in patients with self-reported non-celiac gluten sensitivity after dietary reduction of fermentable, poorly absorbed, short-chain carbohydrates'. *Gastroenterology*, 145(2):320-328.e3.

79. Vernia, P., Di Camillo, M., Foglietta, T., Avallone, V.E., De Carolis, A. (2010). 'Diagnosis of lactose intolerance and the "nocebo" effect: The role of negative expectations'. *Digestive and Liver Disease*, 42(9):616-619.

80. Shahab, L., McGowan, J.A., Waller, J., Smith, S,G. (2018). 'Prevalence of beliefs about actual and mythical causes of cancer and their association with socio-demographic and health-related characteristics: Findings from a cross-sectional survey in England'. *European Journal of Cancer*, 0(0).

81. Schoenfeld, J.D., Ioannidis, J.P. (2013). 'Is everything we eat

associated with cancer? A systematic cookbook review'. *The American Journal of Clinical Nutrition*, 97(1):127–134.

82. Thorning, T.K., Raben, A., Tholstrup, T., Soedamah-Muthu, S.S., Givens, I., Astrup, A. (2016). 'Milk and dairy products: good or bad for human health? An assessment of the totality of scientific evidence'. *Food & Nutrition Research*, 60(1):32527.

83. Ernst, E., Schmidt, K. (2002). '"Alternative" cancer cures via the Internet?'. *British Journal of Cancer*, 87(5):479–480.

84. Johnson, S.B., Park, H.S., Gross, C.P., Yu, J.B. (2018). 'Use of Alternative Medicine for Cancer and Its Impact on Survival'. *JNCI: Journal of the National Cancer Institute*, 110(1):121–124.

85. Gardner, C.D., Trepanowski, J.F., Del Gobbo, L.C., et al. (2018). 'Effect of low-fat vs low-carbohydrate diet on 12-month weight loss in overweight adults and the association with genotype pattern or insulin secretion'. *JAMA*, 319(7):667.

86. Hall, K.D. (2017). 'A review of the carbohydrate–insulin model of obesity'. *European Journal of Clinical Nutrition*, 71(3):323–326.

87. Reidlinger, D.P., Darzi, J., Hall, W.L., et al. (2015). 'How effective are current dietary guidelines for cardiovascular disease prevention in healthy middle-aged and older men and women? A randomized controlled trial'. *The American Journal of Clinical Nutrition*, 101(5):922–930.

88. Hooper, L., Martin, N., Abdelhamid, A., Davey Smith, G. (2015). 'Reduction in saturated fat intake for cardiovascular disease'. *Cochrane Database of Systematic Reviews*. June (6).

89. Huang, T., Xu, M., Lee, A., Cho, S., Qi, L. (2015). 'Consumption of whole grains and cereal fiber and total and cause-specific mortality: prospective analysis of 367,442 individuals'. *BMC Medicine*, 13(1):59.

90. Fung, T.T. (2010). 'Low-carbohydrate diets and all-cause and cause-specific mortality'. *Annals of Internal Medicine*, 153(5):289.

91. Kraut, R., Patterson, M., Lundmark, V., Kiesler, S., Mukopadhyay, T., Scherlis, W. (1998). 'Internet paradox. A social technology that reduces social involvement and psychological well-being?'. *American Psychologies*, 53(9):1017–1031.

92. Lin, L. yi, Sidani, J.E, Shensa, A., et al. (2016). 'Association between social media use and depression among US young adults'. *Depression and Anxiety*, 33(4):323–331.

93. Lup, K., Trub, L., Rosenthal, L. (2015). 'Instagram #Instasad?: exploring associations among Instagram use, depressive symptoms, negative social comparison, and strangers followed'. *Cyberpsychology, Behavior and Social Networking*, 18(5):247–252.

94. Choudhury, M., De Gamon, M., Counts, S., Horvitz, E. (2013). 'Predicting depression via social media'. *ICWSM*, 13:1–10.

95. Woods, H.C., Scott, H. (2016). '#Sleepyteens: Social media use in adolescence is associated with poor sleep quality, anxiety, depression and low self-esteem'. *Journal of Adolescence*, 51:41–49.

96. Carrotte, E.R., Vella, A.M., Lim, M.S. (2015). 'Predictors of "liking" three types of health and fitness-related content on social media: A cross-sectional study'. *Journal of Medical Internet Research*, 17(8): e205.

97. Sidani, J.E., Shensa, A., Hoffman, B., Hanmer, J., Primack, B.A. (2016). 'The association between social media use and eating concerns among US young adults'. *Journal of the Academy of Nutrition and Dietetics*, 116(9):1465–1472.

98. Mabe, A.G., Forney, K.J., Keel, P.K. (2014). 'Do you "like" my photo? Facebook use maintains eating disorder risk'. *International Journal of Eating Disorders*, 47(5):516–523.

99. Bardone-Cone, A.M., Cass, K.M. (2007). 'What does viewing a pro-anorexia website do? an experimental examination of website exposure and moderating effects'. *International Journal of Eating Disorders*, 40(6):537–548.

100. Holland, G., Tiggemann, M. (2016). 'A systematic review of the impact of the use of social networking sites on body image and disordered eating outcomes' *Body Image*, 17:100–110.

101. Valkenburg, P.M., Peter, J., Schouten, A.P. (2006). 'Friend networking sites and their relationship to adolescents' well-being and social self-esteem'. *CyberPsychology & Behavior*, 9(5):584–590.

102. Gonzales, A.L., Hancock, J.T. (2011). 'Mirror, mirror on my Facebook wall: effects of exposure to Facebook on self-esteem'. *Cyberpsychology, Behavior and Social Networking*, 14(1–2):79–83.

103. Chou, H-T.G., Edge, N. (2012). '"They are happier and having better lives than I am": The impact of using Facebook on perceptions of others' lives'. *Cyberpsychology, Behavior and Social Networking*, 15(2):117–121.

104. Vogel, E.A., Rose, J.P., Roberts, L.R., Eckles, K. (2014). 'Social comparison, social media, and self-esteem'. *Psychology of Popular Media Culture*, 3(4):206–222.

105. Vohs, K.D., Heatherton, T.F. (2004). 'Ego threat elicits different social comparison processes among high and low self-esteem people: Implications for interpersonal perceptions. *Social Cognitive and Affective Neuroscience*, 22(1):168–191.

106. Pittman, M., Reich, B. (2016). 'Social media and loneliness: Why an Instagram picture may be worth more than a thousand Twitter words'. *Computers in Human Behavior*, 62:155–167.

107. Becker, A.E., Burwell, R.A., Gilman, S.E., Herzog, D.B., Hamburg, P. (2002). 'Eating behaviours and attitudes following prolonged exposure to television among ethnic Fijian adolescent girls'. *The British Journal of Psychiatry*, 180:509–514.

108. Becker, A.E., Fay, K.E., Agnew-Blais, J., Khan, A.N., Striegel-Moore, R.H., Gilman, S.E. (2011). 'Social network media exposure and adolescent eating pathology in Fiji'. *The British Journal of Psychiatry*, 198(1):43–50.

109. Latzer, Y., Spivak-Lavi, Z., Katz, R. (2015). 'Disordered eating and media exposure among adolescent girls: the role of parental involvement and sense of empowerment'. *International Journal of Adolescence and Youth*, 20(3):375–391.

110. Frederick, D.A., Daniels, E.A., Bates, M.E., Tylka, T.L. (2017). 'Exposure to thin-ideal media affect most, but not all, women: Results from the perceived effects of media exposure scale and open-ended responses'. *Body Image*, 23:188–205.

111. Grabe, S., Ward, L.M., Hyde, J.S. (2008). 'The role of the media in body image concerns among women: A meta-analysis of experimental and correlational studies'. *Psychological Bulletin*, 134(3):460–476.

112. Levine, M.P., Murnen, S.K. (2009). '"Everybody knows that mass media are/are not [pick one] a cause of eating disorders": A critical review of evidence for a causal link between media, negative body image, and disordered eating in females'. *Journal of Social and Clinical Psychology*, 28(1):9–42.

113. Barlett, C.P., Vowels, C.L., Saucier, D.A. (2008). 'Meta-analyses of the effects of media images on men's body-image concerns'. *Journal of Social and Clinical Psychology*, 27(3):279–310.

114. Primack, B.A., Swanier, B., Georgiopoulos, A.M., Land, S.R., Fine, M.J. (2009). 'Association between media use in adolescence and depression in young adulthood'. *Archives of General Psychiatry*, 66(2):181.

115. Madhav, K.C., Sherchand, S.P., Sherchan, S. (2017). 'Association between screen time and depression among US adults'. *Preventative Medicine Reports*, 8:67–71.

116. Stamatakis, E., Hamer, M., Dunstan, D.W. (2011). 'Screen-based entertainment time, all-cause mortality, and cardiovascular events'. *Journal of the American College of Cardiology*, 57(3):292–299.

117. Boepple, L., Thompson, J.K. (2016). 'A content analytic comparison of fitspiration and thinspiration websites'. *International Journal of Eating Disorders*, 49(1):98–101.

118. Tiggemann, M., & Zaccardo, M. (2016). '"Strong is the new skinny": A content analysis of #fitspiration images on Instagram'. *Journal of Health Psychology*, 1359105316639436.

119. Tiggemann, M., Zaccardo, M. (2015). '"Exercise to be fit, not skinny": The effect of fitspiration imagery on women's body image'. *Body Image*, 15:61–67.

120. Holland, G., Tiggemann, M. (2017). '"Strong beats skinny every time": Disordered eating and compulsive exercise in women who post fitspiration on Instagram'. *International Journal of Eating Disorders*, 50(1):76–79.

121. Robinson, L., Prichard, I., Nikolaidis, A., Drummond, C., Drummond, M., Tiggemann, M. (2017). 'Idealised media images: The effect of fitspiration imagery on body satisfaction and exercise behaviour'. *Body Image*, 22:65–71.

122. Chasler, J. (2016). 'Fitspiration: Empowering or objectifying? The effects of fitspiration and self-objectification on exercise behavior'. *Theses Dissertation*. August.

123. Thompson, P.D., Crouse, S.F., Goodpaster, B., Kelley, D., Moyna, N., Pescatello, L. (2001). 'The acute versus the chronic response to exercise'. *Medicine & Science in Sports and Exercise*, 33(6 Suppl): S438–45; discussion S452–3.

124. Tuomilehto, J., Lindström, J., Eriksson, J.G., et al. (2001). 'Prevention of type 2 diabetes mellitus by changes in lifestyle among

subjects with impaired glucose tolerance'. *The New England Journal of Medicine, 344*(18):1343–1350.

125. King, N.A., Hopkins, M., Caudwell, P., Stubbs, R.J., Blundell, J.E. (2009). 'Beneficial effects of exercise: shifting the focus from body weight to other markers of health'. *British Journal of Sports Medicine*, 43(12):924–927.

126. Kemmler, W., Bebenek, M., Kohl, M,, von Stengel, S. (2015). 'Exercise and fractures in postmenopausal women. Final results of the controlled Erlangen Fitness and Osteoporosis Prevention Study (EFOPS)'. *Osteoporosis International*, 26(10):2491–2499.

127. Colcombe, S., Kramer, A.F. (2003). 'Fitness effects on the cognitive function of older adults'. *Psychological Science*, 14(2):125–130.

128. Ströhle, A. (2009). 'Physical activity, exercise, depression and anxiety disorders'. *Journal of Neural Transmission*, 116(6):777–784.

129. Harvey, S.B., Øverland, S., Hatch, S.L., Wessely, S., Mykletun, A., Hotopf, M. (2018). 'Exercise and the prevention of depression: Results of the HUNT cohort study. *American Journal of Psychiatry*, 175(1):28–36.

130. Anglin, R.E.S., Samaan, Z., Walter, S.D., McDonald, S.D. (2013). 'Vitamin D deficiency and depression in adults: systematic review and meta-analysis'. *British Journal of Psychiatry*, 202(02):100–107.

131. Spence, J.C., McGannon, K.R, Poon P. (2005). 'The effect of exercise on global self-esteem: A quantitative review'. *Journal of Sport and Exercise Psychology*, 27(3):311–334.

132. Hamer, M., Stamatakis, E., Steptoe, A. (2009). 'Dose-response relationship between physical activity and mental health: The Scottish health survey'. *British Journal of Sports Medicine*, 43(14):1111–1114.

133. Kilpatrick, M., Hebert, E., Bartholomew, J. (2005). 'College students' motivation for physical activity: Differentiating men's and women's motives for sport participation and exercise'. *Journal of American College Health*, 54(2):87–94. doi:10.3200/JACH.54.2.87-94

134. Hausenblas, H.A., Fallon, E.A. (2006). 'Exercise and body image: A meta-analysis'. *Psychology & Health*, 21(1):33–47.

135. Prichard, I., Tiggemann, M. (2008). 'Relations among exercise type, self-objectification, and body image in the fitness centre environment: The role of reasons for exercise'. *Psychology of Sport and Exercise*, 9(6):855–866.

136. Furnham, A., Badmin, N., Sneade, I. (2002). 'Body image dissatisfaction: gender differences in eating attitudes, self-esteem, and reasons for exercise'. *The Journal of Psychology*, 136(6):581–596.

137. Bamber, D.J., Cockerill, I.M., Rodgers, S., Carroll, D. (2003). 'Diagnostic criteria for exercise dependence in women'. *British Journal of Sports Medicine*, 37(5):393–400.

138. Berczik, K., Szabó, A., Griffiths, M.D., et al. (2012). 'Exercise addiction: symptoms, diagnosis, epidemiology, and etiology. *Substance Use & Misuse*, 47(4):403–417.

139. Phillips, K.A. (2012). 'Body dysmorphic disorder'. *Encyclopedia of Body Image and Human Appearance*. January, 74–81.

140. Thomas, A., Tod, D.A., Edwards, C.J., McGuiga, M.R. (2014). 'Drive for muscularity and social physique anxiety mediate the perceived ideal physique muscle dysmorphia relationship'. *The Journal of Strength and Conditioning Research*, 28(12):3508–3514.

141. Spencer, R.A., Rehman, L., Kirk, S. (2015). 'Understanding gender norms, nutrition, and physical activity in adolescent girls: a scoping review'. *International Journal of Behavioral Nutrition and Physical Activity*, 12(1):6.

142. Ebrahim, I.O., Shapiro, C.M., Williams, A.J., Fenwick, P.B. (2013). 'Alcohol and sleep I: effects on normal sleep'. *Alcoholism: Clinical and Experimental Research*, 37(4):539–549.

143. Walker, M. (2017). *Why We Sleep: The New Science of Sleep and Dreams*. Penguin, UK.

144. Janszky, I., Ljung, R. (2008). 'Shifts to and from daylight saving time and incidence of myocardial infarction'. *The New England Journal of Medicine*, 359(18):1966–1968.

145. Black, P.H., Garbutt, L.D. (2002). 'Stress, inflammation and cardiovascular disease'. *Journal of Psychosomatic Research*, 52(1):1–23.

146. Rozanski, A., Blumenthal, J.A., Kaplan, J. (1999). 'Impact of psychological factors on the pathogenesis of cardiovascular disease and implications for therapy. *Circulation*, 99(16):2192–2217.

147. Black, P.H. (2003). 'The inflammatory response is an integral part of the stress response: Implications for atherosclerosis, insulin resistance, type II diabetes and metabolic syndrome X'. *Brain, Behavior, and Immunity*, 17(5):350–364.

148. Marx, J. (2004). 'Inflammation and cancer: the link grows stronger'. *Science*, 306(5698):966.

149. Chakraborty, A., McManus, S., Brugha, T.S., Bebbington, P., King, M. (2011). 'Mental health of the non-heterosexual population of England'. *British Journal of Psychiatry*, 198(02):143–148.

150. Tabaac, A., Perrin, P.B., Benotsch, E.G. (2018). 'Discrimination, mental health, and body image among transgender and gender-non-binary individuals: Constructing a multiple mediational path model'. *Journal of Gay & Lesbian Social Services*, 30(1): 1–16.

151. Berger, M., Sarnyai, Z. (2015). '"More than skin deep": stress neurobiology and mental health consequences of racial discrimination'. *Stress*, 18(1):1–10.

152. Chong, C.S.M., Tsunak, M., Tsang, H.W.H., Chan, E.P., Cheung, W.M. (2011). 'Effects of yoga on stress management in healthy adults: A systematic review'. *Alternative Therapies in Health and Medicine*, 17(1):32–38.

153. Holt-Lunstad, J., Smith, T.B., Baker, M., Harris, T., Stephenson, D. (2015). 'Loneliness and social isolation as risk factors for mortality'. *Perspectives on Psychological Science*, 10(2):227–237.

154. Holt-Lunstad, J., Smith, T.B., Layton, J.B. (2010). 'Social relationships and mortality risk: A meta-analytic review'. Brayne C., ed. *PLoS Medicine*, 7(7):e1000316.

155. DiMatteo, M.R. (2004). 'Social support and patient adherence to medical treatment: A meta-analysis'. *Health Psychology*, 23(2): 207–218.

156. Kawachi, I., Berkman, L.F. (2001). 'Social ties and mental health'. *Journal of Urban Health: Bulletin of the New York Academy of Medicine*, 78(3):458–467.

157. Uchino, B.N. (2006). 'Social support and health: A review of physiological processes potentially underlying links to disease outcomes'. *Journal of Behavioral Medicine*, 29(4):377–387.

158. Cable, N., Bartley, M., Chandola, T., Sacker, A. (2013). 'Friends are equally important to men and women, but family matters more for men's well-being'. *Journal of Epidemiology and Community Health*, 67(2):166–171.

159. Goddard, M., Smith, P. (2001). 'Equity of access to health care ser-

vices: Theory and evidence from the UK'. *Social Science & Medicine*, 53(9):1149–1162.

160. Watt, I.S., Franks, A.J., Sheldon, T.A. (1994). 'Health and health care of rural populations in the UK: Is it better or worse?' *Journal of Epidemiology and Community Health*, 48(1):16–21.

161. Judge, A., Welton, N.J., Sandhu, J., Ben-Shlomo, Y. (2010). 'Equity in access to total joint replacement of the hip and knee in England: cross sectional study'. *BMJ*, 341:c4092.

162. Newton, J.N., Briggs, A.D.M., Murray, C.J.L., et al. (2015). 'Changes in health in England, with analysis by English regions and areas of deprivation, 1990–2013: a systematic analysis for the global burden of disease study 2013'. *Lancet*, 386(10010):2257–2274.

163. Cutler, D.M., & Lleras-Muney, A. (2006). 'Education and health: evaluating theories and evidence'. *National Bureau of Economic Research*, (No. w12352).

164. Henderson, M. (2017). 'Being on a zero-hours contract is bad for your health'. www.ucl.ac.uk/ioe/news-events/news-pub/jul-2017/zero-hours-contract-bad-for-health.

165. Lundberg, O. (1991). 'Causal explanations for class inequality in health – an empirical analysis'. *Social Science & Medicine*, 32(4): 385–393.

166. Bartley, M. (2005). 'Job insecurity and its effect on health'. *Journal of Epidemiology and Community Health*, 59(9):718–719.

167. Marmot, M., Geddes, I., Bloomer, E., Allen, J., Goldblatt, P. (2011). 'The health impacts of cold homes and fuel poverty, www.friendsoftheearth.uk/sites/default/files/downloads/cold_homes_health.pdf.

168. Krieger, J., Higgins, D.L. (2002). 'Housing and health: time again for public health action'. *American Journal of Public Health*, 92(5): 758–768.

169. Whitelaw, S., Swift, J., Goodwin, A., & Clark, D. (2008). 'Physical activity and mental health: The role of physical activity in promoting mental wellbeing and preventing mental health problems: an evidence briefing'. *NHS Scotland Health*.

170. Crawford, D., Timperio, A., Giles-Corti B, et al. (2008). 'Do features of public open spaces vary according to neighbourhood socio-economic status?'. *Health Place*, 14(4):889–893.

171. Finkelstein, M.M., Jerrett, M., DeLuca, P., et al. (2003). 'Relation between income, air pollution and mortality: a cohort study.' *CMAJ*, 169(5):397-402.

172. Wrigley, N. (2002). '"Food Deserts" in British cities: Policy context and research priorities'. *Urban Studies*, 39(11):2029-2040.

173. Benzeval, M., Taylor, J., Judge, K. (2000). 'Evidence on the relationship between low income and poor health: Is the government doing enough?' *Fiscal Studies*, 21(3):375-399.

174. Stamatakis, E., Wardle, J., Cole, T.J. (2010). 'Childhood obesity and overweight prevalence trends in England: evidence for growing socioeconomic disparities'. *International Journal of Obesity*, 34(1):41-47.

175. Kunst, A.E, Mackenbach, J.P. (1994). 'The size of mortality differences associated with educational level in nine industrialized countries'. *American Journal of Public Health*, 84(6):932-937.

176. Fredrickson, B.L., Roberts, T.A., Noll, S.M., Quinn, D.M., Twenge, J.M. (1998). 'That swimsuit becomes you: sex differences in self-objectification, restrained eating, and math performance'. *Journal of Personality and Social Psychology*, 75(1):269-284.

177. Stapleton, P., Crighton, G.J., Carter, B., Pidgeon, A. (2017). 'Self-esteem and body image in females: The mediating role of self-compassion and appearance contingent self-worth'. *Humanist Psychology*, 45(3):238-257.

178. Bluth, K., Neff, K.D. (2018). 'New frontiers in understanding the benefits of self-compassion'. *Self Identity*, August:1-4.

179. Wasylkiw, L., MacKinnon, A.L., MacLellan, A.M. (2012). 'Exploring the link between self-compassion and body image in university women'. *Body Image*, 9(2):236-245.

Quizzes

Weight bias questionnaire adapted from: Morrison, T.G.and O'Connor, W.E. (1999). 'Psychometric properties of a scale measuring negative attitudes toward overweight individuals'. *The Journal of Social Psychology*, 139: 436-445.

Emotional eating quiz adapted from: Arnow, B., Kenardy, J., Agras, WS. (1995). 'The Emotional Eating Scale: The development of a measure to assess coping with negative affect by eating'. *International Journal of Eating Disorders*, 18(1):79–90.

Body image and media quiz adapted from: Calogero, R.M., Davis, W.N., Thompson, J.K. (2004). 'The sociocultural attitudes toward appearance questionnaire (SATAQ-3): Reliability and normative comparisons of eating disordered patients'. *Body Image*, May 1;1(2):193–8.

Exercise addiction questionnaire adapted from: Szabo, A., Griffiths, M.D. (2004). 'The exercise addiction inventory: A new brief screening tool'. *Addiction Research and Theory*, 12(5):489–99.

Body appreciation scale adapted from: Tylka, T.L., Wood-Barcalow, N.L. (2015). 'The body appreciation scale-2: Item refinement and psychometric evaluation'. *Body Image*, 12:53–67.

Loneliness quiz adapted from: Hughes, M.E., Waite, L.J., Hawkley, L.C., Cacioppo, J.T. (2004). 'A short scale for measuring loneliness in large surveys: Results from two population-based studies'. *Research on Aging*, 26(6):655–72.

ACKNOWLEDGEMENTS

This book has been such a joy to write. It wasn't easy, that's for sure, but I think I enjoyed the process this time more so than with the first one! Naturally there are a few people I need to thank:

Firstly, my amazing family, for being so supportive every step of the way, and dealing with me being super stressed – at least there were no recipe-related breakdowns this time!

To the entire amazing team at Head of Zeus who asked me to write the exact book I was so keen to write. To me this just proves that I couldn't ask for a better publisher. Also to the team at Northbank Talent for believing in me in the first place.

A few special notes: Firstly, Laura Thomas, who has been the most incredible mentor I could have hoped for. If it weren't for you I wouldn't have started down the non-diet path, so I'm so glad you asked me to come on your podcast back in 2016!

Secondly, to my amazing friends in the healthcare space, who challenge my ideas, are always up for an interesting discussion, and who are a constant source of inspiration: Maxine, Anjali, Kimberley, Alan, and CS.

Finally, thanks to Lin-Manuel Miranda for providing the soundtrack to my writing process!

INDEX